Evidence from Within

Evidence from Within

A Paradigm for Clinical Practice

Steven A. Frankel

JASON ARONSON

Lanham • Boulder • New York • Toronto • Plymouth, UK

Published in the United States of America
by Jason Aronson
An imprint of Rowman & Littlefield Publishers, Inc.

A wholly owned subsidiary of
The Rowman & Littlefield Publishing Group, Inc.
4501 Forbes Boulevard, Suite 200, Lanham, Maryland 20706
www.rowmanlittlefield.com

Estover Road
Plymouth PL6 7PY
United Kingdom

British Library Cataloguing in Publication Information Available

Library of Congress Cataloging-in-Publication Data

Frankel, Steven A.
Evidence from within : a paradigm for clinical practice / Steven A. Frankel.
p. ; cm.
ISBN-13: 978-0-7657-0590-7 (cloth : alk. paper)
ISBN-10: 0-7657-0590-7 (cloth : alk. paper)
1. Psychotherapy—Evaluation. I. Title.
[DNLM: 1. Center for Collaborative Psychology and Psychiatry. 2. Psychotherapy—methods. 3. Mental Health Services. WM 420 F8293e 2008]

RC480.5.F694 2008
616.89'14—dc22 2007047373

Printed in the United States of America

∞™ The paper used in this publication meets the minimum requirements of American National Standard for Information Sciences—Permanence of Paper for Printed Library Materials, ANSI/NISO Z39.48-1992.

Contents

Acknowledgments

It makes the most sense to start with my chemistry professors at Amherst College and Bob Dreisbach, my adviser during the year and a half I spent doing research in the Department of Pharmacology at Stanford. They insisted on and taught me scientific rigor, an objective that seemed to slip away during my psychiatric and particularly my psychoanalytic training. Too often the expectation was that we would just "believe" since it was written in the scriptures of the field or came from the lips of a wise, usually old supervisor.

Phil Erdberg, Ph.D., joined with me a few years afterward. He is a kindred spirit, a great thinker, and an impeccable friend. He added the missing rigor, in part through his interest in assessment and his insistence that we make sure our methods and recommendations were "public and replicable." We have co-conducted this project in three steps and have assessed and followed more than 80 people, are writing a book together describing this work, and conduct workshops and consultation groups that in part function as laboratories in which to test and perfect our model. I see Paul Gilbert, M.D., my steadfast practice partner of over 20 years, every other week to talk things over. The members of my current consultation group are crackerjack clinicians and never fail as they teach me about how psychotherapy works. They currently are Susan Collins, Annie Asche, Shira Marin, Barbara Adamich, Jaime Nissenbaum, Dana Kahn, and Nora Webb.

Thanks so much to Art Pomponio, Ph.D., my very wise editor at Rowman & Littlefield, and to the very efficient and generous editorial team with whom I have had the privilege of working, Mary Catherine La Mar and Melissa McNitt.

And my kids. Cara is a just to be licensed child psychologist and tireless in her commitment to finding solutions to human pain and suffering. Peter is an almost fully trained landscape architect and a far clearer thinker than his dad. Tracy, my stepdaughter, will have her Ph.D. in psychology soon, while she and her husband Iishwara are simultaneously producing our grandchildren. And then there is Hilary, my other stepdaughter. Hilary is the artist who created the cover of my last book. She is an absolutely delightful human being—and a smart one!

And, finally, Hilary's and Tracy's mom, Diane. If you need to find the best neuropsychologist, the wisest psychotherapist, and the best friend and wife ever, do look up Diane Engelman, Ph.D.

Introduction

In this book, I will review the most current information about whether psychotherapy is effective, under what circumstances, with which patients, and to what degree. In it, I will take us through the evolution of a method of psychotherapy that we at the Center for Collaborative Psychology and Psychiatry believe can be used by any practitioner in his or her office with the real-world patient population that practitioners see every day. This method has been twenty years in creation. Its development began with the "three-person field" study that Philip Erdberg, Ph.D., and I hatched in the early 1990s, when we first used a psychologist-assessor as a consultant and included him or her as an integral member of the psychotherapy team.

The Controversy

Bringing us to these projects was the realization that the explanation of what makes psychotherapy work is so elusive. Perhaps that observation helps explain why the practice of person-to-person psychotherapy has become so controversial.

Who is to blame for the antitherapy wave of the 1990s? In my opinion, none other than ourselves, the psychotherapists. Especially implicated, I would guess, are psychodynamically oriented therapists, including those that call themselves interpersonal, relational, and existential. Unlike our medical brethren, we are late in our willingness to track and document our results and even place our multimodal diagnostic criteria on firmer, more encompassing ground than is available from the American Psychiatric Association's *Diagnostic and Statistical Manual of Mental Disorders*. The result has traditionally been the rampant, unsupported assertion that psychotherapy, in whatever favored incarnation, works, and outrageous defensive shielding of ourselves from scrutiny. An internist could never, of course, get away with that failure of accountability.

Nonetheless, in spite of the antitherapy and probiology movement of the past 10 or so years, holding that psychotherapists do better with cookbooks prescribing just the right formula for every step of each kind of therapy, there seems to be a renewed consensus even among some of the most hard-core behavioral and biological types. These practitioners concede that psychosocial treatment is at least conditionally effective, that clinical expertise makes at least some difference in whether and how a therapy succeeds, and that contextual factors, most particularly the quality of the therapy relationship, legitimately account for a sizable part of therapy's benefit.

Of course, there are many kinds of psychotherapy with an interpersonal component. Definitions, even within a particular school of thought, tend to be nonspecific, with one type blending into another. Nonetheless, advocates of a particular theory and method can be close to fanatical in denouncing other types of treatment and claiming theirs as the best.

All that said, whatever the value to a psychotherapy of technical orchestration, according to my observations the timing and magnitude of change in a psychotherapy is often not clearly tied to the therapist's deliberate efforts. I am referring to the seemingly impossible moves toward health that occur for the patient in a skillfully conducted psychotherapy of most any denomination. And, indeed, these shifts are often inexplicable. They seem to happen magically, following some hard-to-discern nonverbal map that is likely to be different in each therapy.

Still, for many of the critics of interactive psychotherapies, a formula for treatment, especially if it has been derived from and validated in randomized controlled trials, should be enough. After all, like all medical practitioners, we are scientists, and science strives to understand the true nature of things.

But does it?

Thomas Kuhn (1962), in his enduring book *The Structure of Scientific Revolutions*, traces the way views of scientific certainty have evolved. A parallel in physics was the move from a positivistic Newtonian view of events to quantum mechanics and its focus on the probability that an event will take place and on when and where. His conclusions are unmistakable. Gospel in one era becomes assertion or at least approximation in the next. This shift is paralleled in philosophy by the prominence of postmodernism beginning with German philosophers and sociologists late in the 19th century, such as Burger, Husserl, Heidegger, and Weber. In accord are the moves to modernism and postmodernism in literary criticism (Pinsky, 1976) and to intersubjective, relational viewpoints in depth psychology.

The Projects

Our data from three clinical studies, with the third now in process, conducted with real patients in typical therapy offices, has allowed us to develop the method alluded to earlier in this introduction. Our first two projects each consisted of about 25 patients, many seen over the course of several years and most agreeing to follow up for well beyond 5 years after the completion of treatment. All our patients have received at least part of the assessment protocol of the Center for Collaborative Psychology and Psychiatry, consisting of clinical interviews and psychological or neuropsychological testing. This practice, as integrated into treatment, provides an ongoing corrective for conducting the therapy. As we have evolved our testing, retesting, and monitoring procedures, especially during the past 3 years, they have become more comprehensive. We are now able to follow those protocols on a more regular, albeit flexible case-specific basis during treatment and follow-up. As in my past books (Frankel, 1995, 2000, 2007), in this book several completed cases are discussed in detail.

We have two additional books in mind. In the first, Philip Erdberg and I will elaborate on how we do our work, detailing our continuous integration of psychological assessment with psychotherapy. Through this process, we find our way in a ceaselessly changing psychological and personal environment. In the second book, we plan to present effect sizes and descriptive data from formal diagnostic assessments and reassessments of our work, having by then followed a sizable group of Center patients for several years. Our goal is get ever closer to a picture of what makes psychotherapy work and when and with whom. We will compare our findings to those published in the literature and comment on their statistical, clinical (effectiveness), and research value (efficacy), commenting on the advantages and limitations of office-based data.

The vehicle for the delivery of our services is an association of professionals we call the Center for Collaborative Psychology and Psychiatry. We have trained several groups of therapists in our collaborative assessment and psychotherapy techniques, and in this way we have reached dozens of patients.

This Book

Why is this book necessary? Why not replace interpersonal psychotherapy with behavioral treatments? Are biological treatments not the wave of the future? The answer is that neither is enough. People's behavior is made up of more than cognitive schemas, and, at least at this point, psychopharmacology is only in the early stages of its development, and any psychiatrist can attest to the hit-and-miss quality of psychopharmacological treatments. Moreover, life is just more exciting than all that. Human relationships supported by both thought and emotion are complex. It is a cliché by now that the human mind cannot be fully replicated by a computer. Anyway, who would want it to be? What then would we do about the surprise and discovery that make life and, indeed, psychotherapy so exhilarating and promising?

CHAPTER ONE

Orientation

How certain can a psychotherapist be about the value of the therapy he or she is delivering? Will the treatment be effective, and will it last? Forget the overly technical for the moment. To a point, the question can be boiled down to the simple notion of whether the treatment is working. Progress can be measured and tracked using a variety of tools ranging from the patient's verbal report to self-assessment inventories to more complex psychological tests. So what exactly are we hoping to achieve?

First, we need to target something. But how do you categorize the patient's difficulties, especially since psychological complaints tend to be so personalized? How also do you know what parts of the problem to focus on and in which order? Then we need a reliable and practical method for delivering help and assessing whether it is effective. This line of thinking raises the question of the reliability of your procedures for monitoring progress. And what do you do about the time and cost required to do this work and whether it can be carried out in the office?

Psychotherapy Under Siege?

Psychotherapy, as it has been traditionally practiced, is under siege. As implied in the previous paragraphs, it is frequently criticized as too costly, too inefficient, and generally lacking in clinically cogent and practical means for following change, keeping the therapist accountable for the therapy's outcome. The sad reality is that these allegations are often heavy with truth.

They describe a clinical procedure based in subjectivity and frequently bolstered by assertion. By reference to our projects and the literature on psychotherapy, this book attempts to address these deficiencies. It encourages therapist and patient to ask the hard questions about the nature of treatment: how, if, and when it works. What exactly is psychotherapy? What accounts for therapeutic change? When in the therapy exchange should the therapist act and in what ways (Frankel, 2007)? When, how, and to what extent should psychotherapy be used with a particular patient? What kind of therapy or alternative treatments are most appropriate with a particular patient? What amount and kinds of change are being sought and can reasonably be achieved within the scope of the patient's resources and the therapist's capability? Attempting to grapple with these complexities, this book presents a model for psychotherapy practice that incorporates techniques for planning, orchestrating, and following the changes sought by the patient. These techniques have been selected so that they can be readily used by office-based clinicians.

Yes, in most types of psychotherapy, whether delivered by a psychiatrist or a practitioner without medical training, the patient and therapist interact in a disciplined way, attempting to understand and ameliorate the sources of the patient's distress. When studied meticulously, this interaction can be described, and nodal points bounding change can often be identified and studied (Hilsenroth, 2007; Jones & Pulvos, 1993; Lambert, 2007; Luborsky, 1984; Luborsky & Crits-Cristoph, 1990; Watson & Rennie, 1994; Weiss, 1993). The progression sought may be concrete and easily measured, as when the patient graduates from school or advances professionally, or its character and magnitude may elude objectification. However, limiting these determinations is the personalized nature of the patient's report and the therapist's observations of that change. The fact is that the patient's and the therapist's appraisals are always riddled with subjectivity, biasing their clinical impressions and expectations in the direction of what they would like to find or think they see (for a comparison of this source of error with that associated with formal psychological assessment, see Weinberger & Westen, 2004). It is also difficult to prove that an observed change in the patient is due to, rather than simply correlated with, the work of the therapy. Events in life, developmental influences, and other people's contributions, such as those of family and friends, may have played the greater role in creating the change.

To understand whether and how a psychotherapy is working, none of these factors is irrelevant, making research on psychotherapy a challenging if not ultimately imperfect endeavor. Sorting out this network of interacting influences is the purview of process-oriented research on psychotherapy

(Jones & Pulvos, 1993; Silberschatz, 2005). Its complexity and the probability that its meticulous pursuit would undoubtedly deflect us from our clinical duties, however, makes outcome our criterion for the study from which the observations and recommendations in this book are derived. Outcome also guides us in selecting useful and cost-effective methods of appraising change in therapy.

In all our cases, a second opinion by another clinician, a psychologist-assessor, is obtained as part of our treatment procedure, an arrangement we call "the three-person field." The therapist and patient have access to the psychologist-assessor throughout their work together. In addition to providing formal testing data, this person serves as a consultant to the therapy. In adult cases, the psychologist-assessor routinely administers the following assessment instruments: (a) during the initial assessment and then approximately once every 18 months, the Rorschach and usually the Thematic Apperception Test; (b) every 6 months, the Personality Assessment Inventory, the Symptom Checklist-90 (SCL-90), the Neuropsychological Impairment Scale, and any other tests or self-report inventories, such as the Hamilton or Beck Depression scales, that provide information about problem areas of specific concern for that patient; and (c) a running account of the patient's problems on a biweekly or monthly basis using the brief clinical status checklists provided by the Target Complaint and Goal Attainment questionnaires.

The instruments named have been carefully selected for clinical relevance as well as the accuracy and scope of the information they provide. Our impression is that for most patients, this assessment sequence can be repeated on schedule without creating an undue financial burden and an unwelcome disruption in the therapy. Further, while testing provides diagnostic information and evidence of effectiveness, it is also incorporated in and contributes to the therapy dialogue and is likely to play a part in the changes that result (Finn, 2007; Finn & Fischer, 1997; Fischer, 1994, 2000).

During the initial evaluation and throughout treatment, consultations with specialists are also sought as needed. Any specialty pertinent to the mental health field, including education, psychopharmacology, genetics, neurology, and general medicine, may be enlisted.

Consistent with the author's described paradigm for psychotherapy are the requirements of any thoughtfully practiced medical science. No physician would defend a treatment without clearly articulated criteria for diagnosis and progress. Second opinions are the rule in general medicine. Medical tests and radiological imaging are always used to confirm and expand on a diagnosis. Why, then, have we as psychotherapists been willing to forgo rigorous accountability in our clinical work? After all, the patient's well-being is in our hands and deserves as much attention and respect as when he or she is treated for a medical illness. By incorporating practical ways in which therapist and patient can follow their work and by encouraging them to be meticulous in devising and revising their definition of psychotherapy so that it fits that particular case, the therapist and patient begin to address these deficiencies.

I am not overlooking the fact that most psychotherapists present at least some of their clinical work to a consultant or in case-oriented conferences. In both of these situations, however, the case material presented may not be verbatim or may not capture the nonverbal, contextual dimension of the therapy interaction. More to the point, there is rarely a person outside the therapist and patient who gets to experience the patient directly.

Our Three Projects

Eighty case studies from two earlier projects and already about 30 additional cases from the current one provide the data on which this model has been developed (Frankel, 1995, 2000, 2007). The Center for Collaborative Psychology and Psychiatry, in all its incarnations, was the vehicle for the ongoing development of this practice. The essence of this method, collaborative psychology, was devised by the author and is described in his three books. Collaborative psychology emphasizes the centrality of the authenticity and strength of the therapeutic relationship. In this model, psychotherapy is a two-way process. The therapist and patient provide feedback to each other so that they can readjust their methods and goals as the patient's clinical requirements change.

Introducing a third party, a psychologist-assessor, into the therapy ensures that two perspectives in addition to the therapist's and patient's will continually be available (Finn, 2007; Finn & Fischer, 1997; Fischer, 1994, 2000). These contributions come both from the psychologist-assessor's clinical impressions and from the findings of his or her psychological or neuropsychological assessment. This approach is collaborative from two vantage points. First, the therapist and patient provide feedback to each other, progressively modifying their shared and private views of the key factors in their work. Their impressions are supported by the measures of therapeutic progress provided by the assessment inventories as well as the self-report questionnaires completed separately by patient, family, and therapist. The second level of collaboration is between the psychologist-assessor and the therapist and patient, individually and jointly. Further discussion of this collaborative assessment and treatment method is found in chapter 5.

The Center was designed for the purpose of providing treatment according to this model. We communicate with other centers using similar principles, most particularly the Center for Therapeutic Assessment in Austin, Texas, headed by Stephen Finn, Ph.D., and with the group working with Constance Fischer, Ph.D., professor of psychology at Duquesne University in Pittsburgh, Pennsylvania.

Regarding those involved in this project, Diane Hannah Engelman, Ph.D., is my codirector at the Center. She is trained and certified in neuropsychology and psychological assessment. She has years of experience as a psychotherapist and has a specialty in psychological aspects of medical illness. Philip Erdberg, Ph.D., has been my coinvestigator in all three of these projects. George Silberschatz, Ph.D., has been our trusty consultant. Together with Phil, he contributes his expertise in research design and execution. Phil is also a core associate of the Center. His expertise includes psychological testing, and he coauthored a major book on the Rorschach test with the late John Exner, Ph.D. Paul Gilbert and I are trained and board-certified general and child psychiatrists as well as psychoanalysts. By virtue of training and experience, we, together with Phil, who also has training in psychoanalysis, are well equipped to understand the traditional requirements of in-depth psychotherapy.

What Can Psychotherapy Offer?

Begin with the question of what psychotherapy can really offer. Faith in the process does not mean much when your 10-year-old daughter says that no one likes her or when you find yourself feeling stuck in a marriage or job that feels stale. In these situations, you need results. In both cases, the initial visits to a therapist are likely to be reassuring. After all, if you have done your homework, that person probably came highly recommended and has years of experience. And, at times, we all need reassurance.

Not likely to be apparent at the time of the first encounter are the therapist's personal and professional limitations and biases. How, for example, do you know that he or she will actually deliver? Why in the world, given the little you know about his or her background and personal life, would you trust that he or she is able to empathize with or even understand your dilemma?

Let's say that you are depressed and that the therapist is intolerant of worry and inaction. How well will that therapist comprehend what you need? How impatient will he or she be if you procrastinate about following his or her recommendations? While therapists are generally thoughtful and well intentioned, this one might not believe in the coddling you think you need, or, alternatively, he or she may be too sympathetic for your tastes. In brief, the comforting presence you encounter when you first meet a therapist is likely to cover a personality as complicated and sometimes as private and unpredictable as yours. No doubt, training and discipline help the therapist sift through and regulate his or her responses, choosing those that he or she believes will be most constructive at the moment. Still, interpersonal reliability will at best be a product of a collaborative process in which you and the therapist get to know each other, in some ways intimately. Its limits will be set by such informal factors as the events in both of your lives, the ways you both intuitively gauge and track the therapeutic alliance, and even the way you both feel about fees.

Several sessions later, your absolute certainty about the therapist may begin to wear thin. That's lucky, in a way, since you might instead have spent several months or even years in therapy before taking your doubts seriously.

But, then, maybe it's you. Maybe the therapist is on track and simply pushing you to your limit. Your impression is that he or she is off base, and yet to benefit from this therapy, you may need to tolerate his or her unwelcomed observations. Like in the Ken Kesey novel *One Flew over the Cuckoo's Nest*, it is hard, maybe impossible, to tell who is crazy in a case like this—yourself or the therapist. This dilemma is an old one, elaborated years ago by R. D. Laing (1965) and Thomas Szasz (1961).

Psychotherapy Involves Two Human Beings

Like it or not, connecting with a person, especially when one of them is fragile, requires another human being. To be sure, technical expertise helps, but how does a therapist catch on to the subtle nuances of a patient's problems without major contributions from intuition and empathy? How does that therapist know what to do and say and when to make his statements? And what goes into the elusive quality called clinical judgment?

However, given that the interactive aspect, the human piece, of a psychological or psychiatric intervention can rarely entirely replace the technical, how reliable is the therapist's clinical judgment? What can the therapist promise? The variables predicting the fate of any interaction are complex and interrelated. Among the factors determining the course of a psychotherapy are clinical expertise, empathy, and concern, all at least partially subjective.

For a closer look at these issues, take Dori, who was 26 at the time this story begins. Dori had graduated from an excellent college but after a near debacle in her life was forced to return to her parents' home to work in a temporary job doing clerical work in a large corporation. Following graduation from college 2 years previously, she found work as an assistant account executive at a prestigious advertising agency. At that point, she planned to go on to business school, following in the footsteps of her mother, who was a successful businesswoman.

What a disaster. Uncharacteristically, Dori rapidly became muddled and inefficient in her work, grasping at straws to correct and explain her failures. After 6 months, she was fired from her job and was forced to return to her parents' home in despair, her self-esteem shattered.

Here's where Dori met Thea, a therapist chosen by her mother. Always confident and impressively clad in an expensive suit, Thea was a sure thing. Thea's covert message was clear: listen, follow my lead, and be careful not to think too much. In essence, Thea advocated a system of thought control and meditation. Hungry for relief, Dori complied. And, indeed, she felt better each time she saw Thea. No medication was prescribed.

But Thea misfired. The unwritten rule in that treatment was apparently that Dori never question Thea's authority. Implied was that the wisdom Thea imparted was all that Dori needed to reestablish a healthy frame of mind. Little consideration was given to helping Dori become self-sufficient. For example, Thea never considered having Dori contribute to the cost of the treatment. Thea's fee was shockingly high, but that didn't get questioned either. All these omissions were overlooked by both Dori and her parents since Dori remained in so much emotional distress. Tragically, however, 3 years later, when Dori was ready to enter a doctoral program in public health, she again crashed into a depression, this time worse than the original one. Now it was the fear of again failing that was responsible.

Nonetheless, Dori was intent on going to graduate school. In spite of her near paralysis, she decided to move to a distant city to attend a university that offered her a generous grant. Here's when Dori met Wanda, a psychiatrist who was willing to prescribe medication and seemed refreshingly thoughtful and generous. Right from the beginning, Wanda, who was unmarried and childless, treated Dori like a daughter. Then, when Dori required more time and patience from Wanda as her world seemed to spin out of control, Wanda became punitive. The problem was that Dori was overwhelmed by the fear that she would fail to meet the demands of graduate school and became increasingly dependent on Wanda for reassurance.

In fact, the more anxious Dori became, the more medication Wanda prescribed: at first, Prozac, up to 80 milligrams a day; then Tegretol, stopping at 1,200 milligrams a day; and finally Geodon, building up to 120 milligrams a day. While Wanda was at first sympathetic and even maternal with Dori, she apparently had her own needs that by inference she hoped Dori would meet, hence the ever-increasing dosing of medication, most likely Wanda's way to biologically quell Dori's anxiety and demands. This tension continued to build for months, making Dori feel ever more desperate. Then, finally and sadly, it was terminated when Wanda fired Dori, telling her that she had a "histrionic personality disorder," a problem of a magnitude that Wanda said she would not be able or willing to treat.

At this point, Dori was in her second year of public health graduate school. She lived in a drab apartment in a large city far from her hometown. She was progressively feeling psychologically damaged, unappealing, and, given the hit she had recently sustained to her self-esteem, despairing about ever amounting to anything professionally.

And then, voilà! Suddenly, as if by magic, everything began to change for Dori. This time the initial mover was not a psychotherapist.

Out of necessity, Dori moved to a new, cheaper, but, as it turned out, distinctly friendlier neighborhood. She now had a little extra money to spend and plenty of people in their late 20s to keep her company. Her public health graduate school experience also took a distinct turn for the better. Her courses finally began to capture her imagination.

Ultimately, as critical or even more important to her current sense of well-being than these life changes, is the fact that Dori soon entered treatment with another psychiatrist, this time an intuitively gifted behaviorist. But this therapist seemed to understand Dori and maintained the boundaries Dori required to use the therapy for her own needs. Apart from cutting back on Dori's medications, the psychiatrist made direct and practical recommendations to Dori. While not as emotionally complex as Wanda, this psychiatrist, Dr. Crane, had her feet on the ground. She told Dori enough about her own life to make Dori comfortable but not burden her. Dr. Crane confided, to Dori's relief, that she was happily married and had three children she loved and admired, thus assuring Dori that she had no personal needs for Dori to fulfill through the psychotherapy.

At this point, remarkably, 1 year post-Wanda, Dori is thriving. She has a bevy of friends and has entered an internship in public health, a path that she is confident will lead to an ideal career. She is dating again and is beginning to feel normal for the first time in several years. She speculates that, when she can afford to, she would like to try in-depth psychotherapy. She still hopes that she will find the perfect therapist but knows that such a person may not exist.

Before going on, let's catalog the influences that were instrumental in Dori's more recent progressions and regressions. (a) It is likely that Thea was too unreflective and sure of herself to recognize that she was on the wrong track with Dori. She also missed Dori's need for both antidepressant and mood-stabilizing medication. (b) Wanda, next, took advantage of Dori's search for a caretaker to meet Wanda's own needs. When that misfired, she gave Dori a damning diagnosis and tried to contain Dori's growing desperation with ever-increasing doses of medication. Finally, she fell into an even worse transference–countertransference trap by actually becoming the agent of failure for Dori. This episode repeated Dori's experience at the advertising agency during her first postcollege year, and dismissal from treatment was precisely the outcome Dori most feared. (c) In contrast to miscalculations by two therapists who were sure of themselves, Dr. Crane's reducing Dori's medication, practical suggestions, and appreciation of Dori's age-appropriate need for autonomy were helpful. She directly supported Dori's finding an exciting career track and making friends in a strange city. Dr. Crane was also perceptive. She was the first therapist to make the incisive observation that Dori's success in her career might be tantamount to an assault on Dori's father, who had given up his own promising career to go into business with his own faltering father. She also used cognitive retraining techniques to curb Dori's self-deprecation, which by then had become obsessive. By that time, Dori was plagued with images of becoming a bag lady and could rarely get this prospect out of her mind.

Does Psychotherapy Work?

Why is this the place to start an examination of the literature? Read the up-to-date research on what makes psychotherapy work. The conflicting claims about this subject are neatly documented in the debates in Norcross, Beutler, and Levant's (2006) *Evidence-Based Practices in Mental Health* and in the newest edition of *Bergin and Garfield's Handbook of Psychotherapy and Behavior Change* (Lambert, 2004). These authors, even in their presumably dispassionate reviews of the debates in the literature, may implicitly favor what Bruce Wampold (2001) calls either the "contextual model" or the "medical model" as applied to psychotherapy. In fact, it would seem unreasonable to expect each to be entirely without a point of view and for that bias to be completely absent from his volumes.

The medical model in psychology and psychiatry, according to Wampold (2001), "differs from the medical model in medicine primarily because in psychotherapy the effects due to 'specific' therapeutic ingredients and to incidental, 'contextual' factors are both psychological, creating conceptual as well as empirical ambiguities" (p. 15). Wampold's medical model, as I understand his use of the term, includes all structured aspects of psychotherapy falling under the behavioral heading, from setting treatment goals to prescribing specific interventions, such as the homework and the hierarchical planning of interventions. The complementary model he describes "emphasizes the contextual factors" (p. 23) as they contribute to engagement in psychotherapy. The "contextual factors" cited by Wampold begin most prominently with the therapeutic relationship. Referring to Frank and Frank (1991), he also mentions hope engendered by the therapist, new learning experiences, a sense of mastery created by the therapist's interventions, and the opportunity for the patient to practice new attitudes and forms of behavior.

There is a bewildering assortment of interactive psychotherapies from which to choose. Whatever else each accomplishes, all presumably deliver some form of contextual support. Among them are the traditional Freudians, Freudian dissidents such as Carl Jung (1975) and Melanie Klein (1957), neo-Freudians like Fromm (1970) and Horney (1937), interpersonalists beginning with Sullivan (1953), client-centered therapists, and relational psychotherapists. Generally the theories advocated are based on clinical observation, not hard data (Luborsky et al., 1999). Added to this list are more structurally oriented theoreticians, such as Aaron Beck (1976) and the behaviorists. There are also master clinicians like Marsha Linehan (1993), the researcher-clinician who created dialectical behavioral therapy, who have supported their theories with helpful but limited research.

I suppose the lack of specificity inherent in the contextual model is okay as far as it goes. According to that viewpoint, therapists from most schools of thought should be helpful to their patients if they pay meticulous attention to their personal requirements and are caring. Further, every decent therapist knows that he or she frequently gets results, often results that last. Manualized protocols prescribing standardized interview and remediation procedures just aren't human, and the subject matter that therapists deal with, like it or not, is human. Prominent among the commentaries arguing this point is that by Westen, Novotny, and Thompson-Brenner (2004).

Still, every practitioner, no matter how liberated, also wants objective guidelines and reassurance of achieving results. To this end, there is safety in procedures derived from studies involving randomized controlled trials (RCTs). This experimental condition seeks to give every participant in a clinical trial an equal chance of being assigned to either the control or the treatment category. Meeting this requirement makes it likely that there will be comparability between control and therapy groups and that the findings will be meaningful. One prominent case of practice guidelines developed from research using RCTs is empirically supported treatment (EST) (Chambless & Hollon, 1998; Chambless et al., 1996; Kendall, 1999; Kendall & Schambless, 1998; Nathan & Gorman, 1998), which are defined by the American Psychological Association Task Force on the Promotion and Dissemination of Psychological Procedures (1995) as "treatments shown efficacious in randomized clinical research trials with given populations." The demonstration of treatment efficacy used in the formulations of ESTs usually involves RCTs in which interventions are applied to diagnosed cases and analyzed against a comparison condition, for example, a waiting list or an alternative treatment.

There is every reason to pay close attention to ESTs and their implications for technically improving the practice of psychotherapy. For a typical example of the way ESTs are used constructively, see Maruish's (2002) *Essentials of Treatment Planning*, which leaves plenty of room for clinical judgment even though it is written as a guide for managed care. However, formal research designs employing RCTs also have deficiencies. For example, RCTs typically exclude many of the patients whom clinicians are likely to encounter in their offices since characteristically between 40% and 70% of the applicants are refused participation (Westen et al., 2004), controls may be lacking or inadequate (Lambert, 2004), or the assessment instruments used may be validated and normed on populations different from one's own. Evaluators and judges may be relatively unskilled or biased through their adherence to a particular model of treatment. Measures are often too limited or nonspecific to be clinically very meaningful. Typical is the study of 327 subjects by Beutler et al. (1991), who in spite of their sophistication as researchers, determined outcome of cognitive, experiential, and self-directed therapy using the Beck Depression Inventory, the Brief Symptom Inventory (an abbreviated version of the SCL-90-R), The Hamilton Rating Scale for Depression, the Barrett-Lennard Relationship Inventory, and the Working Alliance Inventory. None of these measures is either broad or deep reaching.

Add to the previously mentioned list of imperfections frequently encountered with RCTs the restrictions in time allocated to follow-up and the lack of adequate controls often reflecting budgetary restrictions. These shortcomings obviously limit the long-term value of such studies. In addition, except for the more qualitative psychodynamically informed studies, formal research on the efficacy of psychotherapy tends to be about treatments lasting no more than 18 months and often for much shorter periods. Moreover, the psychosocial modality used in these studies tends to be limited to cognitive-behavioral treatments (Lipsey & Wilson, 1993).

Follow-up for these studies tends to be carried out for a year or two and only rarely for longer than 5 years (Wampold, 2001; Westen et al., 2004). Limited-duration follow-up may miss the protracted resolution of or exclude reappearances of the targeted condition. Episodes of these generally recurring psychological conditions may repeat over a person's lifetime or at least for substantial portions of it. In addition, pathological entities often change in character over time as, for example, is the case when major depression develops into a bipolar disorder in a person's mid-20s. In part because of these considerations, realistic longitudinal studies with adequate follow-up are difficult and expensive to design and execute.

Moreover, the data obtained on follow-up are generally paltry, consisting of self-report questionnaires, telephone conferences, or a few periodically administered face-to-face interviews at each follow-up. The most widely used self-report inventories for follow-up, such as the SCL-90, consist of a limited range of questions about symptoms. They usually fail to incorporate complex or overlapping symptomatic constellations. In addition, these inventories often cover a range of concerns not accurately reflecting those that the therapist and patient are likely to be focusing on in their treatment.

Roth and Fonagy (2005) discuss the virtues and limitations of different hierarchies of evidence according to their susceptibility to bias. Choices range from RCTs to randomization without controls (as may be found in single-case designs) to cohort studies where groups of patients are allocated to specific treatments. Then there are retrospective studies where patients with similar outcomes are grouped and differences accounted for. Least rigorous are reports using clinical impressions. The authors believe that within this category, single-case studies, where the patient is his or her own control, may become more relevant in time. Single-case studies are convenient to carry out and inexpensive and can be office based. Clearly, the more rigor introduced into the study, the more artificial the treatments offered. The challenge for us and for practitioners in general is to develop ways to optimize treatment to meet a patient's unique requirements without sacrificing flexibility. Research-derived guidelines, such as those contained in ESTs, may do only part of the job. In addition, it needs to be remembered that a patient's requirements often shift throughout treatment, making superfluous an EST that was originally useful (Frankel, 2000, 2007).

In the controversy about the applicability of RCTs and, in turn, ESTs for clinical work, serious doubts are raised about the general applicability of EST guidelines. Witness Stein, Lerer, and Stahl's (2005) representative work, *Evidence-Based Psychopharmacology*. Judging from this volume, much that is currently accepted as standard biological treatment for psychiatric disorders is as yet technically unsubstantiated. Nonetheless, there is no scarcity of ESTs listing when and how to use these drugs in treatment. As one of many examples, I was surprised to learn that lithium carbonate is the only mood-stabilizing drug whose efficacy for mania has been adequately substantiated in clinical trials. Nonetheless, there are a raft of other drugs that are commonly used for the treatment of mania even though they have been subjected to fewer and less definitive studies than lithium. Many, including valproic acid and antiepileptics such as carbamazine, have plenty of support from clinical practice for their value in the treatment of mania. The newer mood-stabilizing antiepileptic lamotragine is also used in the treatment of mania, although it seems to be uniquely effective in the treatment of bipolar depression.

More disturbing are comments such as those by David Healy (2005), a British psychiatrist. He views the reputation for specificity that many psychotropic drugs have earned as products of manipulation by the pharmaceutical industry. He uses selective serotonin reuptake inhibitor (SSRI) antidepressants as an example. His opinion is that the central psychotropic action of these drugs is on anxiety, not depression. Nonetheless, they have been marketed as antidepressants. In addition, except for their side-effect profiles, the SSRIs are no more effective for depression than the older tricyclic antidepressants, and in fact the tricyclics may be more effective than the SSRIs with a subgroup of depressed patients (Nierenberg, 1994; Schatzberg, Cole, & DiBattista, 2005).

In summary, the nature and efficacy of interactive psychotherapy, the identity of who should receive it, the impact of the therapist's training and ideology, and the effect of the sensitivity with which psychotherapy is delivered on outcome are critical areas for research. However, currently, there isn't even a consensus about which modality, medication, behavioral treatment, or interactive psychotherapy is most appropriate for what problems (Pinquart, Duberstein, & Lyness, 2006). This generalization holds for the treatment of most disorders, including those involving "garden variety" depression and anxiety.

Still, the argument between supporters of the contextual model and those who ascribe to the alleged certainty of the medical model and attribute therapeutic superiority to particular pharmacological and interpersonal interventions carries on, and that debate is cogently documented in Norcross et al. (2006), a book that contains a balanced compilation of positions and that reassuringly has been published by the American Psychological Association Press.

Certainly, any temptation to reflexively dismiss procedures derived from randomized controlled trials, such as empirically supported treatment protocols, as too rigid to be clinically applicable or as not representative of ordinary clinical populations is self-defeating (Bohart, 2005; Chambless & Ollendick,

2001; Fisher & O'Donohue, 2006; Hollon, 2006; Hunsley, 2007; Ollendick & King, 2004; Stuart & Lilienfeld, 2007; Wampold & Bhati, 2004). It is hard to imagine that selectively incorporating evidence-based treatments in our procedures would do anything less than augment the nonspecific effects that are always working in a well-executed psychotherapy (Davidson et al., 2003; Goebel-Fabbri, Fikkin, & Franco, 2003; Lambert et al., 2003; Westen et al., 2004). In fact, it makes sense that these measures, when used thoughtfully, should noticeably improve psychotherapy outcome.

Bringing the naysayers and advocates together may be the notion that in spite of adherence to a manualized treatment protocol, a practitioner needs to make his or her own judgment of when and how a particular technical measure should be introduced into a psychotherapy. This judgment is always based on the subjective data of clinical impression tempered by experience and empirical evidence. The evidence I am referring to includes facts about the patient's current life reported by the patient and, at times, other informants; the patient's history, including information about possible genetic factors; a medical examination; self-report questionnaires; and psychological testing. Add to this list the technical information to which the practitioner has access and his sometimes vast clinical experience. Further, in making moment-to-moment decisions, the clinician cannot help but rely on his or her judgment about what the patient can hear and tolerate at any given moment. In this spirit, Sackett et al. (2000) suggest that the "best research evidence refers to relevant research from the basic health and medical sciences, but especially from patient centered research and patient values." They go on to define clinical expertise as including the "(cumulative) ability to use clinical skills and past experience" (p. 147).

It is noteworthy that the relationship between training in the use of treatment manuals and competence in their application needs further study, as does the impact of manualization on the outcome of these treatments as they are carried out in the real world of psychotherapy (Addis, 1997; Addis & Krasnow, 2002; Castonguay, Schut, Constantino, & Halperin, 1999; Kennedy et al., 2004; Levant, 2004). The American Psychological Association's (2002a) criteria for evaluating treatment guidelines fully acknowledges the complex challenge of flexibly meeting a patient's idiosyncratic needs while maintaining the rigorous standards for efficacy and effectiveness that might be achieved through manualized instruction. It is interesting that in two of the few studies on the topic, less experienced therapists appeared more successful at learning to use treatment manuals than more experienced therapists, presumably since they were less set in their ways and less resistant to being retrained (Henry, Schacht, Strupp, Butler, & Binder, 1993; Sandell et al., 2006). By the same token, these therapists might have been less capable of clinical depth than seasoned clinicians. Note that these studies simply need to be regarded as suggestive since each involved a small number of participants and relied on limited data for their conclusions.

As mentioned earlier, a noteworthy alternative to research based on RCTs are single-case designs, potentially conducted by clinicians themselves. This single-participant research (Barlow & Hayes, 1979; Chambless et al., 1998; Morgan & Morgan, 2003) is essentially qualitative, relying on data obtained about a single patient in ongoing psychotherapy rather than from a cohort of patients (Hill & Lambert, 2004). Here the patient is his or her own control, and the work and its outcome are assessed serially. While single-participant protocols are promising for office-based research, needed at this point are designs that clinicians are willing to embrace and use in their offices. To date, most office-based treatment monitoring is restricted to self-assessment questionnaires, and these have limited depth and validity.

Probing the Controversy Through My Own Experience

As a fully trained general and child psychiatrist, with 7 postgraduate years of training in psychoanalysis and a marvelous clinical upgrade at my first job at Children's Psychiatric Hospital at the University of Michigan, I figured I had it down. My work had to be superior to that of lesser trained professionals. How else could it be? After all, for what had I spent those uncountable hours and so much money on tuition, supervision, and missed practice income, anyway?

So let me tell you about my first consultation group and then the second, third, and fourth. In order to expand the reach of the Center, we needed therapists trained in our collaborative model. To begin with, a group of six psychologists, social workers, and marriage and family therapists were recruited. Needless to say, I got to know the work of these practitioners intimately. And I was amazed, completely unprepared, for the lesson I was to learn. These therapists were for the most part mature people who had returned for training after another career or raising children. Almost to a person, they were smart and self-reflective and more than able to seek and hear others' appraisal of their work. They were not inflexibly wedded to theoretical models, as so many of my highly trained colleagues became. And, most important, they strived, asked questions, and generally were impressively successful with their patients.

Most telling about the impact of this experience on me is the before and after. Before this experience, there were only a few select colleagues to whom I would refer. These were mostly people I had worked and studied with over the years. Almost all were psychoanalytically trained or had been heavily exposed to depth psychology. Now, after 4 years, in addition to the original group, I have a bevy of people I trust and can work with clinically. I like, respect, and always learn from them. Of the current group, one is Jungian, another has specialty training in behavioral techniques, and another prefers to work with families.

This testimony appears to support what Norcross, Wampold, and others like them report. Whatever else these psychotherapists delivered, in a general sense they got it right. They were meticulous, caught on to their patient's deeper needs, and most often responded helpfully. Given their different theoretical orientations, their work with patients is a confirmation that the basic requirements for a psychotherapy are human, "contextual" (Wampold, 2001). My first three books examine these interpersonal factors in depth. The rest of what goes into optimizing the results in a psychotherapy, the specific factors as they work with the contextual, is the subject of this book.

Back to Dori

To repeat an earlier point, while several contextual factors affecting outcome in psychotherapy have been identified, I believe that no one is fully clear about exactly how each of these general factors work to effect personal change. That they are important to therapeutic success is intuitively reasonable. But beyond the intuitive, what then? Dori's work with Dr. Crane is a case in point.

Dori knows she was helped by Dr. Crane. But how did Dr. Crane manage to have such a profound impact on her? According to Dori, within a few months of working with Dr. Crane, her mood and confidence lifted beyond her wildest expectations. Apart from changing Dori's medications by eliminating carbamizine and Geodon and lowering the dose of Prozac, what specific factors explain why Dr. Crane succeeded when two other therapists had failed so dismally? Dori says that following the unexpected failure of her psychotherapy with Thea, she learned to be skeptical, to automatically screen expert advice for utility and authenticity. She says that her experience with Wanda was downright traumatic. In contrast, apparently Dr. Crane provided some or all of the general ingredients deemed by Hilsenroth (2007), Luborsky et al. (1985), and Norcross (2002) to be necessary for psychotherapy to work. According to Dori, (a) Dr. Crane emanated reassuring personal attributes, such as warmth and intelligence (the therapist's personal qualities); (b) the therapist–patient relationship with Dr. Crane was solid; (c) Dori was a willing subject (patient qualities); (d) Dr. Crane was apparently sure of herself and was clearly experienced and competent with her craft (the therapist's skill); and (e) Dr. Crane had few overt doubts about the value of the help she offered, yet she could readily incorporate Dori's needs and views with her own so that they made sense to Dori (the therapist's belief in the treatment he or she is providing and its underlying theoretical propositions).

On the side of specificity, Dori says that Dr. Crane knew a lot about managing in a strange city as a young adult. Among her recommendations was that Dori move to a more appropriate neighborhood. Using her cognitive-behavioral skills, she taught Dori practical ways to manage her by now obsessive worries about failure. Added was Dr. Crane's psychologically astute commentary about Dori's unconscious fears of harming her father through her professional success.

But Dr. Crane's skills in the general and specific categories named were certainly not powerful enough to explain how she could have cut so deeply into Dori's despair. Just as a magician pulls rabbits out of a hat, Dr. Crane pulled life out of what at that time was an emptying vessel. There is no doubt that she did it. But how? Apparently, Dr. Crane's inviting Dori to participate in her own thought process, rather than simply insisting that she follow worshipfully as Thea had, was helpful. According to Dori, Dr. Crane is brilliant and perceptive. That she believed Dori could join her in this process and succeed apparently helped set standards for the changes Dori needed to make. Dr. Crane's allowing Dori to prove to herself incrementally that she could do the job probably made the work more convincing for Dori and may have encouraged her to carry on. And then there are the more nebulous qualities called clinical skill and judgment. Apparently, Dr. Crane had plenty of both.

The Bottom Line

Psychotherapy is always a complex mixture of general-contextual and specific-technical factors. Even though comprehension is achieved at one point, therapist and patient still will probably not be certain of exactly how to explain and sustain their success (Frankel, 1995, 2000, 2007). This perspective is consistent with the emphasis on subjectivity of the relational school of psychotherapy (Aron, 1991, 1992, 1996; Hoffman, 1998). It was foreshadowed in the late 19th and early 20th centuries by philosophers such as Heidegger and Husserl (see Smith & Smith, 1995) and sociologists such as Max Weber (see Gerth & Mills, 1946) and Alfred Schultz (see Garfinkel, 1967; Wagner, 1970). This therapeutic stance reflects the hermeneutic, antistructural, antipositivist view that all observations, whether called scientific or not, reflect the observer's subjectivity infused interpretation. It casts doubt on the persistent truth value of any set of observations and the procedures derived from these. From this perspective, ESTs would then be seen as trustworthy for as long as they remained clinically valid in a particular psychotherapy. However, one would not be surprised if they faltered in their ability to guide and predict over time, necessitating that the particular EST procedures be modified or abandoned.

Comprehending how a psychotherapy is working is always elusive. As soon as the therapist—and the therapist and the patient together—achieves clarity about what exactly is troubling the patient and what he or she needs therapeutically, obscurity begins to creep in. The solution to their diagnostic and progress monitoring puzzle, at first seeming to be within reach, begins to fade. The previously mentioned considerations notwithstanding, it would be terribly self-defeating for therapist and patient not to seek to identify the principles guiding their work. This is where the sequential assessment procedure we use at the Center for making diagnostic determinations and monitoring progress comes in.

Making Psychotherapy User Friendly

Lest the reader find this viewpoint discouraging, it would be surprising if the topic of whether reliable guidelines for the practice of a psychotherapy are achievable were less complex and elusive. Understandably, clinicians and researchers seek simplicity and clarity. But just think how dull life would be if the human mind could be reduced to a few concrete, semistable parameters.

Nonetheless, we are faced with the exciting and daunting task of finding a methodology for assessing and monitoring psychotherapy patients that not only works but also can be used by psychotherapists in the offices. It may be worth remembering at the outset that for years people have benefited from psychotherapy, a statement that is supported by the findings of Smith, Glass, and Miller (1980) and Wampold (2001) and the reviews in Lambert (2004). The first step in finding our way within this subjective and technical maze is to explore the issue of making a reliable diagnosis.

A New Paradigm?

My purpose in writing this book and at the Center is to establish a new paradigm for practicing psychotherapy. In this vision, the therapist, of whatever discipline, thinks like a physician. He or she takes responsibility for delivering a therapy that is most likely to be productive and that is not wasteful of the patient's time or money. While fully aware of the human, subjective fabric of our work, he or she is impatient. The patient has come in with an ailment, and the therapist is responsible for fixing it. Knowing the literature really does count since this field is anything but static. Similar is the therapist's willingness to consult with others when he or she reaches the limit of his or her knowledge or when the treatment begins to fail.

The next chapter looks at the research on which factors, specific and non-specific, are likely to be most helpful in conducting a psychotherapy. Then on to the complexities of making a diagnosis and from there to how we do our work with adults and children at the Center. Then to our initial clinical study and our method of delivery at the Center.

Welcome along.

CHAPTER TWO

Assessment in Psychology and Psychiatry: How Similar to Physical Medicine?

Is it possible to eliminate ambiguity from psychosocial diagnosis and treatment? In an ideal world, you could perform radical surgery on the field and make the psychological medical. Every condition would have an empirically supported treatment (EST) protocol.

Here is the way it might look. Begin with the medical. Imagine that you are a medical doctor. A patient comes to you. You begin by establishing a diagnosis using a physical examination, medical tests, and consultations from specialists. Clinical judgment would never be absent from this process. As data became available, you would develop a medical treatment plan, always discussing it with the patient and soliciting his or her input and agreement. Finally, you would carefully and regularly monitor treatment—its progress and failures. And, of course, you would follow up, perhaps for years.

Does the cancer reappear? In what form? How to beat it this time? How can you and the patient arrive at an acceptable level of confidence about the nature of the problem, and how can you attack it at each point during treatment? Will the plan hold and prove reliable?

Or perhaps it is not so clear cut. Take Nathan, a 76-year-old inveterate cigar smoker, with high standards and a crackerjack mind. He built and then, 10 years ago, sold his technology firm and made a fortune. Serious minded, fact oriented, and always precise, Nathan had one Achilles' heel. He tended to develop stomach and bowel problems, including diarrhea and constipation. Always fair, Nathan was never sure whether these symptoms were caused by his body or his mind.

Nathan religiously went to doctors, always receiving logical answers but never in the end being cured. It was the same when he began to feel weak on awakening and noticed that his gait was unsteady. After several missed diagnoses by well-regarded medical doctors, the culprit was finally identified. Whether he liked it or not, Nathan had Parkinson's disease. So, several experts later and after much time and expense, Nathan had his diagnosis.

Nathan's Symptoms Were Explained (or Were They?)

What about his bowel symptoms and even aspects of his weakness? Up to a point, they could conceivably be symptoms of early Parkinson's disease. However, weakness is unusual as a presenting symptom of Parkinson's. And there were other possible explanations as well.

One was entirely psychological and favored by Nathan. Nathan's father died of colon cancer at age 76, and Nathan had been dreading his 76th birthday for years. And he was now 76. Nathan said he missed his father terribly and had always thought about how fitting it would be if he could sign out before he reached the age of his father's demise. Sorry, I know this example is beginning to sound like the kind of psychoanalytic thinking that was so dominant in the 1950s, physical symptoms equaling somatic manifestations of a fantasy or fear. Yet it may be. In fact, even now, 2 years after the first appearance of Nathan's weakness, the matter remains unresolved.

Nathan's Parkinson's has worsened. He is weaker but not because of afflictions of the muscles involved in Nathan's first complaint of weakness. His bowel symptoms are about the same, but he worries about them more as his body begins to fail. His spirit is also flagging, suggesting that he is slipping into depression.

Back to the question of precision. Nathan's medical doctor is seasoned and wise. He was and is baffled. I am Nathan's psychiatrist. Both of us get pieces of the puzzle and are confused by other parts. The physical examination helps, as do medical tests that for the most part have served to rule out other medical entities since few tests, biological or radiological, are diagnostic for Parkinson's. Both of us would like more certainty, but we keep losing our way.

What is the difference between the diagnostic and therapeutic challenge in medicine and in the psychosocial sphere? As we have seen with Nathan, the requirements of both treatment modalities, medical and psychosocial, are conceptually similar, but the technical issues are quite different. Generally, in a psychosocial treatment, you have a patient who complains of an ailment, but even if he or she has physical symptoms, it is the subjective or interpersonal that are targeted, not primarily the physical. In physical medicine, the bias is toward the physical.

No doubt medical complaints always have a subjective component. But when someone is seeking medical care, his or her subjective experience is often of secondary interest to the physician, who, after all, is in practice to treat physical ailments. In contrast, treatments for psychological and psychiatric disorders focus on the patient's anxiety and suffering. Once physical causes are ruled out, the mental health professional is hard pressed to know which components of the patient's personality or environment are most implicated in creating his or her problems. A collaborative dialogue with the treating person helps refine the diagnostic picture. That person can use psychological and neuropsychological testing as well as the clinical impressions of the psychologist-assessor who administers the tests to arrive at a diagnostic formulation of the patient's problem, as we do at the Center for Collaborative Psychology and Psychiatry. The findings even then, however, are rarely definitive. Rather, the product of testing and clinical judgment is likely to be a layering of opinion, only partially of hard facts.

Even psychological testing data may not fully describe a patient's dilemma. The psychosocial practitioner's recourse then is to closely follow the patient both clinically and with the kind of monitoring procedures we use at the Center. In fact, this course of action is most consistent with clinical reality since it is rare for the patient's symptoms and even personal circumstance not to change, at times radically, during a successful treatment. In fact, if the therapy works and problems begin to resolve or shift, one would expect the treatment to take just this course.

The opposing case, suggesting that certainty can be introduced into psychosocial assessment and treatment, is currently being made by practitioners and researchers who are fervent advocates of ESTs (alternatively called empirically based practice) and are dedicated to putting mental health on par with medicine (Kihlstrom, 1998; Kihlstrom & Kihlstrom, 1998; Strauss & Kaechele, 1998; Tanenbaum, 2003, 2005).

Moving to treatment, consider Parkinson's disease again. One knows a lot about the antiparkinsonian drug Sinemet for treating an afflicted patient's shuffling gait and tremor. In contrast, the response to a selective serotonin reuptake inhibitor antidepressant when used to treat depression is much less predictable. Further, in depression, once the symptoms begin to abate, what do you do about the patient's problematic personality or the lack of an adequate support system for maintaining his or her new level of functioning?

But, then, how truly different is it with the medical diagnosis and treatment of Parkinson's given its multiple etiologies and the well-known fact that its course is unpredictable? Complicating the picture further is the observation that emotion may affect the course of Parkinson's and vice versa. In addition, tracking the disease requires the patient's subjective report. Further, this discussion entirely leaves out the personality and the biases of the doctor who, for example, may be so wedded to a particular outcome that he or she misjudges the patient's actual condition. It follows and yet may seem remarkable that according to the available research, the accuracy of assessment in physical medicine and mental health are frequently equivalent (Kubiszyn et al., 2000; Meyer, 2001, 2003; Meyer et al., 2001). In both situations, the actual treatment decisions ultimately rest on clinical judgment.

Consider Keith, a 70-year-old man whose polycythemia was exacting its toll through bone marrow failure. Polycythemia is a cancer of the bone marrow in which red blood cells multiply out of control. The result is weakness caused by the inability of the red blood cells to effectively transport oxygen and ministrokes due to clumps of these cells clogging small arteries. The medications used to treat polycythemia, including a type of interferon, themselves exact a toll. Finally, over years, polycythemia converts to leukemia, as it was doing in Keith.

Keith, who had always been a model of self-reliance, grew to understand and tolerate his condition. He was grateful for the 21 years he had been able to live with his disease. While not particularly self-reflective, he welcomed our weekly talks about the meaning of his life and his impending death.

Everything was set for Keith to say good-bye. In fact, on one Sunday, he gathered his four children and wife around his bed and did just that.

That's when Dr. T. stepped in and spoiled everything. Keith and Dr. T. had been sailing buddies. Dr. T. was a researcher who was an expert in diseases of the bone marrow. He had cared all along for Keith medically and had done all he could to help Keith survive. Dr. T. also was a scientist and took on Keith's case as a challenge. When he caught on to the fact that Keith, his wife, and myself were helping Keith to manage dying, he paradoxically took on the role of prolonging Keith's life with even greater vigor. His by now zealous quest was supported by Keith's two daughters, who resented their stepmother's influence with their father.

Alarmed, I begged Dr. T. to let Keith die peacefully. But he would not hear of it. Since by then Keith was in a rehabilitation hospital close to Dr. T.'s office and quite distant from mine, I progressively lost control of the situation. After convincing Keith that his life could be sufficiently prolonged, Dr. T. introduced progressively more radical medical procedures that at times required rehospitalization for weeks at a time. Over the next 6 months, Keith's health deteriorated, and he slipped progressively into dementia. I had no choice then but to sit by helplessly and watch Keith and his wife suffer as Keith lost track of his intention of dying gracefully. His desperation, as he lost control of his mind, legs, and bowels and bladder, eludes description.

In the end, we all agreed. We had been impressed by Dr. T.'s medical expertise but were appalled by his unreflective heroics. His actions, rather than seeming to be caring as they originally did, emerged as shortsighted and egocentric.

How then might a psychosocial technique emphasizing contextual factors but combined with the principles of a data-focused medical model look?

A Practical Framework

Maruish (2002) does just this as he lays out a manualized model of treatment for a contemporary office-based psychotherapy practice. However, unlike some others who advocate the use of ESTs to guide treatment, he leaves plenty of room in his recommendations for the patient's personal needs and preferences. He is also clearly respectful of the central place of clinical judgment and therapist–patient collaboration in creating a case formulation and treatment plan.

According to Maruish's scheme, first, when working up a new patient, comes the clinical interview. The objective is to see why the patient has come and at this particular time. He recommends a semistructured interview for which he provides a reasonable outline. He includes judgments of functional impairment, personal style, social supports, readiness to change, and, among other categories, the patient's strengths, not just difficulties. Treatment goals are formulated collaboratively by the therapist and patient and, when relevant, third parties. Recommendations are partially structured around the patient's reported and inferred motivation to change. He discusses the use of self-report inventories and psychological testing in creating a case-specific formulation and treatment plan. He advocates treatment monitoring based on the selected treatment goals and using checklists such as the Behavioral Symptom Inventory and the Brief Psychiatric Rating Scale as well as psychological testing to the extent to which their use is practical and affordable.

Since this manual is meant for managed care settings, the assessment instruments Maruish discusses are, for the most part, inexpensive and easy to administer. Consequently, the information they provide about the necessarily complex psychology of the patient and his or her changing requirements and progress is limited. Once again, the responsible clinician is thrown back on the bedrock of clinical judgment. As used by an experienced clinician, this judgment is probably more reliable than would seem obvious given its subjectivity.

While the relationship between clinician experience and treatment results is not a perfect one, the role of clinician training and experience remains unsettled, and the subject continues to be an important aspect of psychotherapy research. Nonetheless, it is hard to imagine that experience and the resulting capacity to make educated clinical judgments could be extraneous to outcome (Addis, 1997, 2002; Alberts & Edelstein, 1990; Castonguay et al., 1999; Levant, 2004; Roth & Fonagy, 2005; Wampold & Bolt, 2006).

Reflecting on the good sense of Maruish's recommendations, it seems remarkable to me that assessment protocols of this sort tend to be followed so inconsistently by psychotherapy practitioners. While I have no hard evidence, my impression is that cutting corners in the use of formal assessment is the rule in clinical practice, with self-report inventories and psychological testing being omitted even when the tests used are bare bones in time and cost. As compared to the distinctly more extensive testing we use at the Center, "bare bones" seems an apt designation for Maruish's protocol. Maruish's format is admirable, especially as compared to assessment as usual. However, since the amount of diagnostic and prognostic information is so much greater from the Center workup, the "bare-bones" approach of even Maruish's scheme may, in fact, may be an example of the mental health community being forced to be penny wise and pound foolish.

Yet my impression is that psychotherapists, except for those advocating time-limited measures, behavioral treatments, and psychopharmacology, have lacked the discipline and, at times, the motivation to be as accountable for the accuracy of their work as are most medical doctors. Regarding motivation, these omissions no doubt make it more comfortable for those of us in practice since no one except the patient is looking over our shoulders. Yet I believe that this lack of accountability is fundamentally inexcusable, especially if we as a discipline want to remain credible to the rest of the professional world.

Returning to Nathan and Keith, where in the dilemmas and ambiguities we encounter in our work does our craft lose its edge to hard medicine? My claim is that the difference is largely qualitative. In physical medicine, regardless of the seeming objectivity of the data guiding the assessment and treatment, the treating person is continually influenced by personal, subjectively guided, clinical judgment and issues involving patient compliance. Further, in general medicine as in psychotherapy, the treatment usually needs to be repeatedly reevaluated and redirected by both participants so that it remains technically and interpersonally accurate. Influencing medical doctor and patient and almost always creating ambiguity are debates among experts about which treatment approach is best (Degury, 2003; Phillips et al., 2001). We have a medical diagnosis for Nathan, but the atypicality and shifting nature of his symptom picture still prevents both the medical and the psychiatric experts from arriving at a comprehensive explanation of his condition. In Keith's case, the sought-after medical expert who insisted on taking over his case knew how to treat only the disease, not the person. In the end, Dr. T. only made matters worse for Keith.

Do I have a right to dismiss blood tests and scans so casually, placing them on a level of utility equal to psychological tests and clinical observation by a psychologist or psychiatrist? In taking this position, am I not unreasonably devaluing medical tests, such as platelet and red blood cell counts and indices, in following and treating Keith's polycythemia? Regardless of statistical evidence putting psychological testing on par with medical tests (Meyer et al., 2001), no one really believes that the reliability of the data from both is equivalent. But look at Nathan and Keith. The point is not numbers versus personality variables. It is, instead, the incredible complexity and often shifting nature of both medical and psychiatric conditions. I'm afraid that when God made both the brain and the body, she didn't intend either to be particularly easy to read or treat in isolation from one another.

Diagnosis

In spite of all the effort invested in creating the major psychiatric diagnostic and statistical manuals—the *Diagnostic and Statistical Manual of Mental Disorders* (*DSM*) in all its incarnations and the 10th edition of the *International Classification of Diseases*—these diagnostic systems remain imperfect. (Krueger, 1999; Krueger & Piasecki, 2002).

Psychiatric entities tend not to be discrete, in contrast with the "categorical" approach taken in the *DSM*. Further, as encountered in clinical practice, many of these entities are subacute, causing vague, elusive discomfort. Then there is the fact that, especially in our area, comorbidity is the rule, depression, anxiety, and compulsive behavior overlapping, for example. Further, patients come to us with particular strengths. Some are well educated and accomplished, some have the capacity for personal reflection and are particularly good at working with a therapist, and some have family and friends to assist them. The *DSM-IV* axis IV rates a patient's "psychosocial and environmental problems," and axis V provides a "global assessment of functioning." These indices help to fill in the picture, but people and their circumstances may change from week to week, and, perhaps more important, their personal assets differentiate them, sometimes markedly, from others.

Speaking to the same issue of accuracy of diagnosis, it is no wonder that Millon (1996), a psychologist and a member of the *DSM* task force, states the following in his widely used book *Disorders of the Personality: DSM IV and Beyond*, "Personality disorder is a dysfunction in person's capacity to cope with life's difficulties" (p. 9). He goes on to say that personality disorders are not disease entities. These disorders "represent deeply embedded and relatively enduring templates of imprinted memories, attitudes. . . . Once psychic structures are in place they are difficult to transform or uproot" (p. 10). He clarifies, saying that personality contains "multiple data levels including biological, humanistic, behavioral, socio-cultural" (pp. 11–12). These levels are "not linear but sequentially interactive and multiply distributed throughout the system" (p. 13). He then points to the relationship of these organizations of data to the systems model and how using them requires "real world clinical decisions," the parameters of which are often neither neat nor simple; "personality disorder can be assessed but not definitively diagnosed" (p. 15). He adds that the systems perspective is always more realistic than a simple diagnostic category. As I read Millon, he holds that the multiaxial *DSM* system is in the right direction but that, in the real world, traits and symptoms are not necessarily consistent over time, there are individual differences in how they are expressed, and people usually do not fit neatly into the diagnostic categories.

Millon makes an additional critical point. When in practice do we as clinicians ever encounter a patient whose presenting symptoms are not influenced by the patient's character? In the least, symptoms and character are intimately connected, with the personality aspects determining and coloring which symptom picture the patient develops. According to Millon (1996), the interaction between *DSM* axis I and axis II is complicated. One can predispose to the other, each interacting with the person's vulnerabilities to influence his or her further development (Maser, Kaelber, & Weise, 1991; Sroufe, Egeland, Carlson, & Collins, 2005). As an illustration, Millon gives the example of the devastating and often immutable effect of a schizophrenic episode on a person's self-esteem. The same, of course, can be said for a serious depression or even a devastating economic reversal. It is hard to imagine anyone emerging from any of these experiences unscathed, remaining as optimistic and unworried as they once were.

Incidentally, in *DSM-IV*, as in *DSM-III*, the thresholds for personality disorders are based on the subjective impressions, the consensus, of the task force that formulated the *DSM* (Morey, 1988). According to Phil Erdberg (personal communication, 2007), there are two other issues. The first, referring to Hurt, Reznikoff, and Clarkin (1991), is "homogeneity," meaning that the system of choosing a diagnosis by selecting a critical mass of constructs in naming a disorder often lumps together very different types of individuals. For example, for the diagnosis of paranoid personality, seven different types and levels of distrust are named, some consistent with normal moodiness. The patient receives the diagnosis if he or she has four of these. The second, referring to Skodol (1988), is "overlap," or one category running into another.

In support of the contention that *DSM-IV* may obscure as well as clarify a psychiatric diagnosis, Roth and Fonagy (2005) say that "the fixed nature of *DSM* categories excludes large groups of heterogeneous patients and people whose pathology is below the threshold for the DSM diagnoses" (pp. 487–488). They state that 30% to 50% of the patients seeking help for mental health problems cannot be diagnosed using the *DSM* because their problems are "subthreshold." Add to this indictment Beutler et al.'s statement quoting Maruish (1999) that "the diagnostic label does not allow the clinician to select among cognitive, interpersonal, or relationship psychotherapies. The symptoms that determine diagnosis are quite insensitive to qualities and characteristics that determine how well prospective patients will respond to them. . . . Most clinicians realize the weaknesses and limitations of diagnosis and develop a large and rich array of treatment possibilities as they seek extra-diagnostic information. . . . This information is consolidated into both a patient formulation and a treatment plan" (pp. 82–83).

Returning to Dori from chapter 1, there is little doubt that she was depressed, qualifying her for the *DSM* diagnosis of major depressive disorder. Bringing in Millon's points about the pervasive effect of character on diagnosis, however, what can we say about Dori's personality? She was obviously characterologically compliant. For example, she asked few questions about her mother's expectations that Dori follow in her career. Similarly, in psychotherapy, she slavishly complied with her first two psychotherapists, although their advice was consistently harmful to her. For example, she took the medications Wanda prescribed for her even though all of them were being overprescribed and in Dori's growing private opinion were probably contributing to her depression. In fact, her inability to make her own judgments became even more troubling for Dori than her depressions.

Millon advocates taking a systems approach to creating a diagnostic formulation. To continue with our exercise, the social systems implicated in the cause and maintenance of Dori's problems were several. For example, there was religion. Dori parents were practicing Catholics. Dori had attended a Catholic high school and was trained to be compliant with authority. Family tradition and expectations also contributed. In Dori's mother's family, female children were expected to enter their mother's profession. The areas missed altogether by all of Dori's therapists except Dr. Crane were those associated with Dori's strengths, with their inevitable contributions from Dori's biological endowment. Given a chance to think and work by herself, Dori quickly revived and thrived on her own.

How then do we now regard Dori's original diagnosis: depression? Certainly she was depressed, but was it the type of biologically based depression described as major depressive disorder in the *DSM*? Dori's depression responded well and independently to judicious medical and psychosocial management. Dr. Crane's advice obviously helped. So did a change of environment. Further, how much of Dori's original presentation can be explained simply by the developmental stress of leaving her family and embarking on her own life? In addition, how much did the persistence of Dori's difficulties reflect improper therapeutic management by both Thea and Wanda? And what about the contribution of a damning misdiagnosis, with Wanda's labeling Dori with a histrionic personality disorder making Dori feel "washed up as a human being?"

Our Expanded Diagnostic Framework

Since we are not working with research subjects but rather with real patients who somehow showed up in our offices, we need to be cognizant of all aspects of their needs and personalities, including their capabilities, the influence of family and culture, their support systems, and the resources they can and are willing to allocate to working out their problems. In contrast, in formal studies carried out in the current research atmosphere using randomized controlled trials, research subjects are characteristically chosen so that they meet the requirements of a particular study. As mentioned in chapter 1, a remarkable 40% of perspective participants are frequently excluded from such studies (Roth & Fonagy, 2005). The outcome measures to be followed are usually carefully defined and selectively targeted as well. As previously discussed, the magnitude and length of the trials and follow-up are typically measured in months, not years, and the assessment instruments used tend to be symptom oriented and self-report in nature.

I have designed the following diagnostic framework with the goal of making it more inclusive than its *DSM* counterpart. It takes into account, for example, temperamental and sociological factors not incorporated in the *DSM-IV*. Also considered are the patient's strengths, often reflected in his or her personal and professional attainments. I have placed at the end of each section, marked with an asterisk and bracketed, a selected list of assessment instruments that might be used to diagnose and track that category. My objective is to describe a real person, accounting for his or her full complexity.

The Diagnostic Framework

The diagnostic framework can be organized as follows:

I. Troubling psychologically expressed symptoms or behavior

(a) Symptomatic

1. Includes all *DSM-IV-TR* axis I disorders as well as milder and more general symptoms interfering with patient's life, such as depression expressed as dysphoric mood or lethargy, a tendency to obsessively worry whether or not qualifying for the *DSM* diagnosis of obsessive-compulsive disorder (OCD), and apprehension whether or not amenable to the *DSM* diagnosis of anxiety disorder.

2. Combined diagnostic disorders such as obsessionality qualifying for the *DSM* diagnosis of OCD but with co-morbid depression or anxiety, disturbances of mood that also qualify for the diagnosis borderline personality disorder, and thought disorders of a complex nature with or without delusions or hallucinations and with subtle mood abnormalities but only marginally qualifying for the diagnosis of schizoaffective disorder.

[*Self-report inventories including the Symptom Checklist-90. Outcome Questionnaire 45, the Personality Asset Inventory, and the Minnesota Multiphasic Personality Inventory. All projective tests including the Rorschach and the Thematic Apperception Test (TAT).]

3. Disorders primarily affecting self-esteem and self-cohesion.

[*All projective tests (more recently dubbed "performance-based personality tests") including the Rorschach and TAT. Others, such as the Adult Attachment Projective, may require training not completed by most psychologists.]

(b) Behavior reflective of personality disorder

1. Chronic, behaviorally expressed conditions manifest as character. These syndromes range from addictions to conduct disorders (for a full discussion of this topic, see Millon, 1996).

[*Scale of Interpersonal Problems, Scale of Psychological Capacities, self-report measures for children and adolescents such as the Behavioral Assessment System for Children (BASC).]

(c) Trauma-based disorders not necessarily qualifying for the DSM *diagnosis of posttraumatic stress disorder, including unresolved childhood trauma manifest as proneness to depression, anxiety, or problematic behavior in adulthood.*

[*Trauma Symptom Inventory.]

II. Adjustment

1. Areas of resilience and strength, including inherent talents, and constructive temperamental traits, such as optimism or the capacity for self-assertion and self-reliance. Studies of the origin of this kind of resilience in childhood and its course throughout life include Block and Block (1986, 1988); Hamilton (2000); Sroufe et al. (2005); Thomas and Chess (1980); and Yates, Dodds, Sroufe, and Egeland (2003).

2. Vocational and avocational accomplishments.

3. Personal goals, including difficulties and successes encountered in achieving these.

4. Current and past relationships, their number, duration, depth, and reciprocity.

[*The Adult Attachment Projective, the TAT, and Robert's Apperception Test (for children and adolescents).]

5. Unwelcomed environmental demands such as those associated with a professional crisis or new developmental requirements, including those connected with aging.

[*There are many. Examples include the 16 Personality Factors, the Scale of Psychological Capacities, the Rorschach, the TAT, the Robert's Apperception Test (for children and adolescents), and the NEO Personality Inventory—Revised (NEO-PI-R).]

III. Neuropsychological

1. Aberrant development in cognition, emotion, and interpersonal functioning. These entities are classed as pervasive developmental disorders in *DSM-IV-TR* and include the autism spectrum ranging from Asperger's syndrome to frank autism as well as congenitally and genetically based developmental delays and retardation.

[*These tests are too numerous and specialized to list here.]

2. Intelligence and deficits in specific areas of cognition.

[*The Wechsler Abbreviated Scale of Intelligence provides a basic screen. A much more extensive battery, the Wechsler Intelligence Tests for either adults or children, provides a great deal more information but takes much more time to administer and score. Educational psychologists have a variety of specialized tests to assess learning difficulties available, as well.]

3. Disorders of attention, memory, perceptual-motor functioning, and processing of cognitive and emotional information. More specifically, these domains of neuropsychological functioning include global cognition, attention, executive functioning, learning and memory, verbal/language function, and visual-perceptual-spatial realms.

[*The decision about which tests to use is complex. However, most of the relevant tests are included in the Neuropsychological Flexible Battery.]

4. Disorders of organization and planning (executive functioning).

[*Decisions about which tests to use is complex. Most are included in the Neuropsychological Flexible Battery.]

5. Problematic aspects of temperament such as proneness to anger or passivity.

[*Scale of Interpersonal Problems and Scale of Psychological Capacities.]

6. Other disorders involving regulation of mood and behavior (dyscontrol syndromes), not classed with personality or pervasive developmental disorders.

[*Personality tests mentioned previously, including the Rorschach and self-assessment behavioral scales, including the BASC and NEO-PI-R.]

IV. Resources and Culture

1. The capacity for and interest in self-reflection and change

[*Scale of Psychological Capacities and Rorschach.]

2. Support systems and financial resources

3. Other problematic conditions based on a dysfunctional family system or the inability to meet cultural expectations

Returning to the Medical Model

Apparently, relative certainty about the nature of a condition and its optimal treatment is often as difficult to achieve in medicine as it is in the practice of psychotherapy. Yet there are differences. The path at least appears to be less well demarcated in the psychosocial area. The variations in the treatment challenges we psychotherapists encounter and in possible creative solutions are unlimited, and the element of surprise, even revelation, is ever present.

However, in effect, we as therapists are all medical practitioners since we have the patient's welfare and future in our hands. While always striving toward objectivity, the therapist's responsibility is to make a thoughtful assessment, take charge of the therapeutic work, monitor its progress, and include the patient as a full collaborator. The treatment strategy adopted needs to be broad enough to include a range of diagnostic entities and flexible enough to allow the therapist and patient to identify and adjust to changes in the patient's requirements as the therapy continues. Ways of monitoring shifts in diagnosis and treatment progress should always be built in.

At times, patients who come to us do not have the financial resources to fully utilize our services. Insurance most often does not pay for outpatient psychotherapy services. In these situations, we as practitioners have two choices. We can refer the patient for treatment by others. Often these referrals are to a less expensive, less highly trained mental health professional or clinic than ourselves. Alternatively, we can labor with the patient to see if we can find a relatively affordable yet efficacious alternative to the version of psychotherapy we would optimally like to provide.

Here, then, has been our challenge as we have carried out our work and studies. Our goal has been to design treatments based on diagnostic procedures that are public and replicable. Replicable means that what we recommend can be reproduced by others. Our assessment techniques need to be not only available to others but of interest to them as well. Public refers to the requirement that our data be transparent enough so that they can be readily understood and used by other practitioners and researchers. From a practical viewpoint, our work needs to be effective, meaning that we have the means (in this case, assessment measures) to be confident in our diagnostic findings and our recommendations. Ease of use also counts since our procedures need to be willingly adopted by therapists for their office practices.

It was with these conditions in mind that we carried out our projects and have evolved the service component of the Center. We have trained a cadre of excellent practitioners to assist us in carrying out our mission. All are skilled in orchestrating the assessment, monitoring, collaborative treatment, and follow-up procedures we have evolved and refined through the Center. They are thoroughly comfortable acknowledging their uncertainties and searching for answers. They are prepared to evolve creative solutions as they encounter the patient's psychological limitations, lack of resources, and absence of real-world support.

CHAPTER THREE

Integrating General and Specific Therapeutic Interventions

It is currently fashionable for biologically and behaviorally oriented practitioners to debunk the value of treatments with a relational focus, especially when these are not evidence based (for an example of this kind of critique, see Ollendick & King, 2004). Psychodynamic, interpersonal, and existential psychotherapies are especially targeted for these criticisms since they rely so heavily on nonspecific, contextual factors, such as the therapeutic alliance, for their effect. Replacing these more traditional approaches in research studies and in empirically supported protocols are designs that are almost exclusively behavioral and pharmacological.

In this chapter and in concert with Norcross, Beutler, and Levant (2006); Lambert (2004); Wampold (2001); Smith & Glass, 1977; and Smith, Glass, and Miller (1980), I take the position that interpersonally informed psychosocial treatments can indeed be powerfully effective for creating symptom relief and personality change. However, in conflict with the tone with which the named authors discuss psychotherapy, I add two qualifications. First, it is intuitively unlikely that specific interventions, tailored to a particular patient, should have as little influence on therapeutic change as Wampold (2001) and Norcross et al. (2006) suggest. Second, the power inherent in the therapist's contextual, interpersonal role can misfire and even harm. Unfortunately, this result happens more often than we might like, as it did in Wanda's work with Dori. Therapists often justify what they do by citing their particular theory, whether dialectical behavioral or Jungian, for example, or by substituting their credentials for humility and even substance. In my opinion, each instance reflects a misapplication of the therapist's authority (Aron, 1996; Frankel, 2007; Grossman, 1996; Hoffman, 1998; Mitchell, 1998).

Further, I add that there is no reason why psychosocial treatments should go unexamined in spite of the inconsistency introduced by the twists and turns encountered as therapist and patient move along. It is our opinion that these treatments can be as readily monitored as those that are behaviorally oriented or pharmacological. With this statement, I am making the claim that psychosocial treatments can be subjected to empirical standards for validation that are as rigorous as those currently used for behavioral or pharmacological treatments. Here I have named a major component of our mission at the Center for Collaborative Psychology and Psychiatry. For the past 10 or so years, we have been engrossed in developing technology for making psychosocial treatments public and replicable. Office-based practitioners can readily use this technology. Our hope is that practitioners will adapt our recommendations, establishing a new paradigm for practical, office-based psychotherapeutic treatment.

I have already noted in chapter 1 that good longitudinal studies in our field are rare. The plethora of conflicting claims about which psychosocial and pharmacological interventions work best muddy the scientific waters. Formal research studies are done using highly selected cohorts of people, usually not equivalent to office-based patient populations. Since mental disturbances may recur over a lifetime, the most useful studies of intervention success often require years to complete. Challenging also to the relevance of these studies is the fact that the character of a treatment invariably evolves over months or years as the patient and his or her needs change. Considering the inconsistency that these shifts introduce, it may be that strict research criteria cannot be maintained as a treatment remains true to clinical requirements and that single-case designs will grow in relevance for studying office-based psychotherapies. Take heart, though. The confounds introduced are no different in physical medicine. Practicing in that discipline with its laboratory tests and radiological scans often just looks more scientific.

Now to the data. Specific treatment measures, whether behavioral or pharmacological, can be used alone, together, or in concert with a relationship-centered psychotherapy to treat disorders of mental health. Apparently, combining a psychosocial intervention and psychopharmacology is often associated with outcomes that are superior to using either alone. In some cases, as when antidepressant medication is used for the treatment of major depression, pharmacotherapy can be effective with or without personal guidance or formal psychotherapy, although few practitioners would choose to exclude these modalities since at minimum they provide monitoring and encouragement. In contrast, behavioral techniques alone seem to be exclusively successful in treating a few conditions, such as isolated phobias (Ghaemi, 2002; Roth & Fonagy, 2005; Stein, Lerer, & Stahl, 2005; Westen et al., 2002).

Elaborating on these statements, in some cases, such as bipolar illness, pharmacotherapy is clearly the treatment of choice (Ghaemi & Hsu, 2005; Roth & Fonagy, 2005). With other diagnostic entities, such as major depressive disorder, neither type of treatment has yet been clearly shown superior. However, in situations like these, it often, if not usually, seems judicious to combine both pharmacological and psychosocial treatments (Pinquart, Duberstein, & Lyness, 2006; Roth & Fonagy, 2005). In fact, in the treatment of bipolar disorder, a collaborative relationship with a psychotherapist and patient education are apparently instrumental for facilitating remissions and patient maintenance (Reiser & Thompson, 2005; Roth & Fonagy, 2005).

There also are cases where psychotherapy and pharmacotherapy seem capable of producing equivalent results. Witness the monograph on the treatment of depression commissioned by the American Psychological Association (Hollon, Thase, & Markowitz, 2002). These authors cite numerous studies showing that cognitive-behavioral therapy (CBT), interpersonal therapy (IPT), and a variety of other treatments produce initial results comparable to those from medication. Over 3 years of posttreatment follow-up, monthly IPT sessions did not maintain the patient as well as continued treatment with high doses of medication. The authors ultimately recommend long-term IPT and CBT maintenance along with continued pharmacotherapy. Conclusions have been similar for the outcome of the major study of treatment for depression by the National Institute of Mental Health (NIMH) (Elkin et al., 1989). Notably, in this massive project, by 18 months posttreatment, the outcome for specific psychotherapy was indistinguishable from that using a well-constructed placebo. Subsequent studies (see Hollon et al., 2002) found that 16 weeks of IPT or CBT could not compare with the efficacy of a continuous course of medication. There were additional data, however, that extending short-term psychotherapeutic interventions by several months substantially improves outcome. That finding led the authors of that article to conclude that empirically supportable treatments that include both psychosocial and pharmacological components are most likely the optimal versions of these treatments over time.

In concert with the data just cited, Roth and Fonagy (2005) state in their concluding chapter that medication and psychological therapy offered alone are often broadly equivalent in their outcomes. While "cessation of pharmacological treatment is often associated with relapse . . . patients are more likely to maintain their gains" when they are receiving psychosocial treatment as well (p. 493). Given the data they have collected, the authors also conclude that "combination treatments (pharmacological together with psychosocial) appear to be more helpful than one or either modality offered alone." Their "observations suggest that patients are likely to benefit when both psychological and pharmacological modes of intervention are available" (p. 493).

My impressions are similar to Roth and Fonagy's. It is hard for me to imagine that the monitoring, support, and structure gained by including a psychosocial component as part of the intervention strategy would not be critical to therapeutic success, even if biological- and cognitive-based interventions are emphasized. As a practicing clinician, it is of particular interest to me to note that in the NIMH depression study, over the longer term psychotherapy and pharmacotherapy were equally effective and that the combination of the two was judged to be superior to either alone. Of course, as with all the other studies I describe, the NIMH study, while massive, was anything but definitive. What I am struck by is that this finding is so consistent with informal impressions from my own clinical experience. For better or worse, we are stuck with the fact that our patients are people: complex, hardly predictable biological organisms powered by the illogic of emotions. Clinical experience consists of exposure over time to these personalized, seemingly unsystematic ways of being that become familiar to the clinician only through his or her own life, work, and empathy (Healy, 2005).

In addition, there is little evidence that the brand of psychotherapy delivered (Lambert, 2004; Smith et al., 1980; Stiles, Shapiro, & Elliot, 1986; Wampold, 2001), whether Freudian, Jungian, or behavioral, makes much of a difference in outcome. Behavioral methods are the psychosocial modality that have been most studied in clinical trials because, I infer, they are structured; easiest to understand and reproduce and thereby favored in contemporary literature (Plunkin, 2006). By inference, from the reports summarized in the sources cited, as well as Lambert's (2004) excellent summary of psychotherapy research, what seems to matter most to psychotherapy success are intangible factors, such as the psychotherapist being fully committed to and competent in his or her craft and consistent in its delivery. The patient needs also to be a willing collaborator, believing in the skill and wisdom of the therapist (Hilsenroth, 2007; Norcross et al., 2006). According to Lambert (2004), "Decades of research have not produced support for one superior treatment or set of techniques for a specific disorder" (p. 167).

And, yet, I have just contradicted my earlier opinion based on experience and intuition that specific interventions tailored to the patient must be capable of making a substantial difference in outcome. This seeming discrepancy can be reconciled only by the idea that each treatment needs to be designed for a specific patient and that the therapist and patient be guided competently through clinical judgment, trial and error, and, if possible, well-timed and well-executed psychological assessment. Ideally, studies of this kind of intervention, probably requiring single-subject research designs (Campbell, 2004), should be carried out to substantiate my claim that specific interventions can be selected or created so that they substantially influence outcome.

Case Vignette: Gary

My experience with Gary, a 47-year-old, socially isolated single man whose story will be developed further in chapter 4, illustrates the kind of clinical flexibility to which I am referring. The pressing therapeutic issue during my first few months as Gary's psychiatrist was dealing with his fury at my challenging his chronic inaction. Within weeks, he had moved from liking my somewhat informal style to reviling me for "lack of professionalism" and wasting his time with my "useless" opinions. His repeated threats to quit treatment each felt like an invitation for combat. He had won all previous wars and annihilated at least six psychiatrists. The last two decided that Gary was a latent schizophrenic and suffered from some unidentified developmental disorder in addition to showing the features of a borderline personality disorder with which he was originally diagnosed.

Once I met his challenge, Gary's magic pill, in addition to dynamically informed interpersonal psychotherapy with me, was dialectical behavioral therapy (DBT), a combination of behavioral and dynamic psychotherapy techniques accompanied by group didactic sessions. This modality was actually suggested by Gary's parents, who, out of desperation, had joined an organization dedicated to providing support for parents of children with emotional illness. Dialectical behavioral therapy seemed promising because measures in addition to conventional psychotherapy and mood-regulating medication were required for Gary to achieve some perspective about his appalling behavior. I am referring to the unmitigated arrogance that alienated just about everyone who came into contact with Gary and explained the resignation of several of his previous therapists. Dialectical behavioral therapy is especially geared for emotionally labile patients, many of whom qualify for the axis II diagnosis of borderline personality disorder from the *Diagnostic and Statistical Manual of Mental Disorders* (4th ed.). The DBT therapist is encouraged to set clear limits, albeit in an empathic manner, and to seek consultation during the treatment since working with this type of patient is usually so trying. In keeping with this diagnosis, Gary characteristically moved from threats of suicide to rage at yesterday's best friends and his remarkably patient and attentive parents for their alleged failings and then always to arrogant self-righteousness in his dealings with me.

Progressively added to our repertoire of interventions were meetings between myself and Gary's parents and a full neurological and neuropsychological work-up. Of course, Gary knew about and had to approve of my meeting with his parents. Then, since I suspected that the bipolar condition Gary was being medicated for did not exist and that he was capable of a far better adjustment than he was used to, I referred him for neuropsychological testing and a neurological examination. As part of the neurological work-up, he was given an MRI and a PET scan of his brain.

Each component added to treatment improved its effectiveness: DBT, the meetings with Gary's parents, my holding firmly to the position that we needed to have expectations for Gary's psychotherapy, and the medical and neuropsychological work-up. Based on my observations and Gary's thoughtful retrospective testimony, behavioral measures have provided reasonable instruction in successful coexistence with others and managing the usual social and logistical demands of life. Being in a group has provided invaluable social feedback for Gary, who for years protected himself from emotional injury by social isolation. Gary was also helped to recognize maladaptive patterns in thinking and behavior when he reviewed confusing or painful experiences in psychotherapy and with his DBT group soon after they occurred (Linehan, 1993). The group also provided him with a framework from which to build the structure and planning functions so absent from his life. Finally, he credits mood-regulating medication for aiding his emotional stability.

As I suspected, except for confirming his already known borderline personality disorder characteristics, Gary's personality and neuropsychological testing were normal. A major finding from these assessments was that his compromised ability to withstand life demands were built largely on myth and the cognitive dulling effect of excessive medication. The intervention required was a reduction in the antipsychotic and sleep medication he had been receiving for years and progressive confrontation with evidence of his considerable personal strengths.

My point in providing this case example is that no single intervention is likely to adequately address a patient's complex needs. Nor could I have told from the outset what measures would be required for Gary to progress. Certainly in Gary's case, slavish adherence to a particular school of therapy or empirically supported treatment (EST) procedure would have compromised my ability to make sense out of and respond to his requirements. With Gary, adherence to a treatment formula by his previous therapists, two of whom were psychoanalysts, had fated him to receive improper medication and unproductive dynamically oriented psychotherapy. It assured him that he would be labeled chronically disabled and that he would conduct his life accordingly.

My solution for finding one's way within the psychotherapy quagmire is quite simple. It is summarized by the single word *humility*. There is absolutely no reason for any therapist to insist on the objectivity of his or her clinical judgment about what will unequivocally help the patient.

I believe that the same principles apply in general medicine. It is only that the medical practitioner has available a physical examination together with laboratory tests that include visualizations of affected areas using scans and X-rays. While ultimately not always more reliable, such data are more uniformly concrete and familiar than the diagnostic information from clinical observation and psychological assessment that we ordinarily have as psychotherapists. In addition, medical data tend to attract less skepticism than psychological data. Surprisingly, however, the validity of the two kinds of data may be equivalent (Meyer, 2003; Meyer et al., 2001, and the extensive bibliography therein). This assertion, as counterintuitive as it might be, has statistical support. Where the Meyer et al. study fails, however, may be in its source in meta-analyses. The rigor of this report begins to fall off with the authors' qualification that the treatments studied had not been carefully matched for the type and quality of research methodology used to study them.

Had I acknowledged to myself that even an orthopedist's opinion is steeped in judgment, I think I would still be able to jog. Instead, when I developed a knee injury 10 years ago, I too readily accepted my orthopedist's recommendations as if they were based in fact rather than opinion. The orthopedist and I had a long-standing, friendly relationship. I trusted him to do his best to preserve the activity I considered the mainstay of my emotional and physical well-being: jogging. I had jogged and run competitively every day of my life since age 14. So I asked very few questions when he insisted on removing a sizable section of the right medial meniscus from my knee rather than resecting a small torn flap from it. He seemed so sure of himself. I asked the usual preliminary questions, read, became aware that major resection was controversial, but eventually felt sheepish continuing to question him. Inexplicably, I worried that he might be critical, even contemptuous of me, if I pushed my uncertainty further. I might not continue to qualify in his mind as a "clear-minded" doctor like himself.

My position about what works in psychotherapy and how to optimize it is that the factors that Wampold (2001) calls "contextual" and that Norcross et al. (2002) call "general," the relational and nonverbal exchange between therapist and patient, make up the necessary part. But I also hold that these elements are not in themselves sufficient to create the best therapeutic outcome. Specific behavioral, medical, and psychologically guided interventions have to count. Of course, these need to be judiciously selected, applied in an affirmative therapy context, and geared meticulously to the patient being treated.

Research on Psychotherapy

Studies of psychodynamic psychotherapy should be promising since such therapy focuses on the details of the therapeutic interaction (Wallerstein, 1992). Disappointingly, however, to date these studies have relied mostly on inadequately supported assertions about whether it works, with whom, and when. The parameters being measured have tended to be unclear. Definitions of what constitutes psychotherapy or psychoanalysis as well as therapeutic change have generally been vague and arbitrary, precluding rigorous comparisons of the outcome data from individual studies. As Bachrach, Galatzer-Levy, Skolnikoff, and Waldron (1991) make clear in their report to the American Psychoanalytic Association, psychodynamically oriented studies are generally poorly designed, even if they have been painstakingly constructed, and they are therefore difficult to compare. As a group, they have tended to be inconclusive. In fact, not all analytic therapists believe that such studies are even possible. Representing this perspective, Stephen Mitchell (1997) discounts the value of psychotherapy research as research since, in his opinion, subjective bias always contaminates the findings.

Other studies of the efficacy of psychotherapy have major limitations. As previously discussed, the contemporary solution to searching for reliable ways to characterize and structure psychotherapy and, within economic bounds, to study it has become to make it time limited, to substitute therapists with limited clinical experience and training, and to replace interpersonal psychotherapy with manualized treatment focusing on medication and behavioral techniques. Empirically supported treatments are introduced to objectify psychosocial treatment and put it on par with general medicine. They may also be intended to simplify and streamline treatments, making them more replicable, appropriate, and affordable for formal research (Crits-Cristoph, Wilson, & Hollon, 2005; Tanenbaum, 2003, 2005; Norcross et al., 2006; Westen & Bradley, 2005; Westen, Novotny, & Thompson-Brenner, 2004). In addition, alarmingly, because of financial realities, there is progressively less incentive for researchers to move beyond studies supported by drug companies—or managed care organizations—from which to base guidelines for treatment.

A good example of these compromises seems evident in the study by Addis et al. (2004), where 80 patients with the diagnosis of panic disorder were studied. All were drawn from a managed care population. The study was designed to distinguish the efficacy of panic control therapy versus treatment as usual. Instruments used to evaluate the therapy included the Beck Depression Index, the Outcome Questionnaire-45, the Panic Disorder Severity Scale, the Fear Questionnaire, and a less well known instrument called the Treatment Credibility Questionnaire. All these instruments are brief and self-administered. Laudably, therapy sessions were audiotaped, and a random sampling was also tested to see if and how the therapists' work deviated from what the author calls "panic control therapy." However, treatment consisted of one to seven sessions completed within 8.5 months. Longer-term outcomes were not assessed.

Similarly, Jones and Pulvos's (1993) sophisticated article compared the outcome of 32 time-limited CBTs for 14.4 weekly or biweekly sessions using the Beck Depression Index, the Depression scale of the Minnesota Multiphasic Personality Inventory, and the Automatic Thoughts Questionnaire, an inventory measuring subjects' habitual negative thoughts. The psychodynamic treatment group received an average of 15.8 sessions. There were two striking differences between the patient groups and the way they were handled: the outcome of the psychodynamic group was assessed with different instruments than the cognitive-behavioral group, namely, the Symptom Checklist-90 and the Brief Psychiatric Rating Scale. In addition, all the participants in the psychodynamic group were not designated depressed as they were in the time-limited behavioral therapy group. In fact, the psychodynamic group was judged to be less troubled than the cognitive-behavioral group, and rather than bear a diagnostic label, they qualified for the study simply because it was felt at intake that they could benefit from brief psychotherapy. Further, half the cognitive-behavioral group was also treated with tricyclic antidepressant medication. So why would you do a research study that compared apples and oranges and then, to add insult to injury, try to make statistical sense out of the result (Sharpe, 1997)? Moreover, surprising about this article is its lack of detail about determining factors in psychotherapy, especially considering Jones's sophisticated contributions to psychotherapy process research technology.

General Factors Required for Psychotherapy to Work: My View

Regarding the general factors with the strongest influence on therapeutic success, Wampold (2001) cites the therapeutic alliance, the therapist's "allegiance" to a therapeutic approach and "adherence" to it as he works, and therapist competence and experience as examples of the "general" factors positively influencing therapeutic outcome. To this list, the contributors to Norcross (2002) add empathy, positive regard, and genuineness including a warm acceptance of the patient; congruence, a factor that includes the therapist's "willingness to be freely and deeply himself" in the therapy and to "convey his personhood" to the patient; repairing alliance ruptures; self-disclosure that is clearly of a personal nature; feedback to the patient; the sensitive management of countertransference, including all the therapist's reactions to the patient; and interpretations in the therapy that are relationally based.

Supporting the opinions expressed by these authors are numerous studies. Several projects demonstrating a relationship between treatment alliance and therapy outcome are reported by Hilsenroth (2007), including those conducted by himself and his colleagues. In his own work, he was interested in this correlation in relation to a collaborative therapeutic assessment process. A typical example of one of these studies is the project reported on by Barber et al. (2000), who found that the therapeutic alliance predicted the outcome of psychotherapy for 86 patients as measured by the Beck Depression Inventory. Subjects received between 16 and 52 once-weekly sessions of manual-guided supportive-expressive dynamic therapy. These investigators found, as had others, that the early alliance was a good predictor of a continued strong connection between therapist and patient as well as response to treatment. In line with these findings are the data from the uncharacteristically large NIMH Treatment of Depression Collaborative Research Program (Elkin et al., 1989; Ogles, Lambert, & Sawyer, 1995), which found clinically significant improvement in all treatment groups, including those receiving clinical management and imipramine (an older, tricyclic non–selective serotonin reuptake inhibitor antidepressant), interpersonal therapy, cognitive-behavioral treatment, and placebo. Outcome measures included the Beck Depression Index, the Hamilton Rating Scale for Depression, and the Hopkins Symptom Checklist 90. A similar set of findings was reported by Krupnick et al. (1996) for a subgroup of patients from the already cited NIMH depression study. The investigators in this study wanted to see the correlation between the therapeutic alliance and psychotherapy outcome. Note that it was the patient's contribution to the alliance, his or her active involvement in the treatment, that was statistically significant in this study, not the therapist's. Parenthetically, I am aware of such an association from my own clinical work.

Alliances can take a variety of forms. Defects can be masked by superficial compliance, for example. The pivotal contribution of the patient's determination to make the therapy work was recently reiterated by 31-year-old Terry, a remarkably bright college graduate who is recovering from a manic attack. In retrospect, Terry is clear that his progress in our work was slowed because his father had been so generous in paying his medical and living expenses since his breakdown. In Terry's words, "I just got lazy. Dad paying my expenses kind of allowed me not to face the reality of my illness and how difficult it would be to lick it."

Regarding correlations of improved outcome with specific interventions, the surprise is that there are so few studies that rigorously confirm such an association. One wonders how this is possible given the attention that randomized controlled trials (RCTs) are receiving and the implications these have for ESTs and empirically based practice. Barrowclough et al.'s (2001) British study is one of several exceptions, advocating CBT above supportive counseling. Adding uncertainty, however, is that each of these studies has its own size or design limitations. By specific interventions, I am referring to psychotherapy techniques with a formal structure, such as those associated with CBT.

Each school of psychotherapy has its own diagnostic criteria and treatment techniques. Freudians focus on instinctual conflict and ego development, Jungians on the healthy development of the self, and interpersonal and relational psychoanalysis on subjectivity. Roth and Fonagy (2005) help resolve the specific-versus-contextual puzzle by restating Norcross's (2002) and Wampold's (2001) position that "although therapy types have an influence on outcome, they do not account for much of the variance in outcome, and that all successful psychotherapies share many common factors" (pp. 50–51). However, Roth and Fonagy note that the majority of psychosocial therapies qualifying for these studies were cognitive-behavioral. They amend this statement by saying that research involving CBT may simply have gotten a head start and that evidence about the effectiveness of other types of therapies will emerge over time. The study by Ogles et al. (1995) noted previously is a case in point since in that very large study, all treatment groups did equally well. In addition, of some interest is the study by Castonguay et al. (1999), where they demonstrated that 30 outpatients who completed treatment of 14 weeks of cognitive-behavioral treatment with or without medication showed results that correlated positively with the therapeutic alliance and the patients' emotional involvement with the therapy. However, in that project, unique aspects of cognitive therapy correlated negatively with outcome at the end of treatment. In this study, the authors inferred that the increased focus on the impact of distorted cognitions seemed to worsen alliance strains, thereby interfering with therapeutic change. Outcome in this study was assessed according to the Beck Depression Index and the Hamilton Rating Scale for Depression as well as the Global Assessment Scale.

When the nonspecific therapy factors cited are in place, conditions are set for the shared, mutually creative state of mind I call "therapeutic conjunction" (Frankel, 2000, 2007). However, the notion of a therapeutic conjunction partially eludes definition since it is neither a concrete entity nor a fixed state. In addition, conjunction in psychotherapy is always building and degrading. As hard as one tries to capture and reproduce this uniquely heightened state of mind, it begins to slip away in the next therapeutic moment. In fact, this elusiveness is part of what is so intriguing about therapeutic conjunction and perhaps the potential of human beings to join together in a way that is therapeutic altogether.

Still, it behooves us to do our best to identify all the factors that optimize psychotherapy. As mental health professionals, we are dealing with people who have come to us asking for help, wanting the benefit of our expertise. While the research has failed to conclusively show that any specific factor such as therapy type overshadows general factors in making psychotherapy succeed, the research does not identify therapies in which an excellent conjunctive frame is in place before specific techniques are applied. By conjunctive frame, I am referring not just to a good alliance and mutual commitment to the therapy work. The requirement, instead, is a uniquely creative, mutually respectful joining of therapist and patient for the common goal of resolving the patient's difficulties and enhancing the quality of his or her life.

However, as good "doctors" of whatever discipline, I think we will agree that in most cases, to treat best, you must have not only a tuned-in patient but also the right technology and techniques for addressing specific treatment issues.

I am most interested in and persuaded of the critical role that contextual factors play in each psychotherapy and, for that matter, in each medical treatment (Frankel, Quill, & McDaniel, 2003; Institute of Medicine, 2001; Inui & Frankel, 2006; Mischler, 1979, 1984; Mischler & Clark, 1989; Najavits & Strupp, 1994; Phillips & Andrews, 2001; Stewart et al., 2000). However, it is incumbent on us as practitioners of a medical discipline to explore specific technical interventions assuming that, as in the case of using the right medication, they can make all the difference in optimizing the results of a therapeutic intervention. Incidentally, not all therapeutic maneuvers are essentially interactive. Some, for example, are educative. Others may involve environmental manipulation undertaken for the patient's benefit.

Specific psychotherapy techniques include CBTs; DBTs; desensitization techniques; treatments for posttraumatic stress disorder, including eye movement desensitization and reprocessing; cognitive structure building and rehabilitation; personal instruction from life coaches and, for that matter, athletic coaches; spiritual instruction; and guidelines for living found in self-help books. Therapy group participation is compatible with some systems of psychotherapy. Added to this list are medication and other biological treatment measures, including transcortical stimulation and electroconvulsive therapy. Note that different types of specific therapeutic interventions may be indicated for different age-groups and diagnostic categories and that cultural considerations may influence therapy choice.

As in playing a musical duet, timing and having a "good ear" are everything in psychotherapy. Add the critical, apparently legitimate role that bedside manner and the placebo effect (Beach & Inui, 2006; Epstein, 1995; Frankel & Gerrity 2007; Frankel & Inui, 2006) play in all treatments. If the integrity of the therapeutic alliance and associated therapist–patient qualities are so important, then probably also is the timing and manner of introducing such technical measures as self-revelation by the therapist, medication, psychological testing and retesting, and revisions of treatment goals and the steps in attaining them. Add the potentially reassuring effect of note taking, including the ongoing gathering of information using, for example, the Target Symptom and Goal Attainment inventories to keep track of the patient's difficulties. At the Center, in addition to our in-depth assessment and monitoring procedures, we use several self-assessment tools selected for the patient's age and presenting problems. We also ask that the patient or parents initially complete a lengthy history questionnaire, a measure that generally contributes to their conviction that we want to know as much as possible about them.

To make sure that I was at least aware of the range of possible specific therapeutic interventions, in initiating these studies I returned to the study of general medicine, neurology, pharmacology, and radiological methods. I was struck by how out of date I was, for example, with newer developments in biochemistry and molecular genetics as these bear on psychopharmacology. It was of no matter that I had actually majored in chemistry in college, concentrating on physical chemistry, or that I had also done the equivalent of 2 years of research in pharmacology. With the help of my wife, who is a neuropsychologist and is proficient in the full range of available assessment instruments, and our consultants, Drs. Erdberg and Silberschatz, I also learned all I could about psychological assessment and its validity and reliability, adding research design and statistics to the mix. In addition, I did my best to train myself to understand the varieties of behavioral therapy. In case it sounds like an overwhelming undertaking, it actually has become the most exciting project of my career, allowing me, within my capability, to discover so much more about the big picture of medicine and psychology, all parts of which bear on what we do at the Center.

The research on psychotherapy, including delineation of specific factors contributing to therapeutic outcome, is assiduously summarized by Roth and Fonagy (2005) and Norcross et al. (2006). The sheer bulk of studies is intimidating, and above that is the problem of comprehending the validity of each and how they relate to one another. What one is immediately struck by is that, except for establishing that nonspecific factors make a difference and through meta-analyses of the findings deriving the effect sizes of those differences, so much has not been definitively studied.

For example, as already mentioned, it appears that interpersonal intervention for major depressive disorder generally is more effective than placebo and that the value of psychotherapy may be equivalent to that of pharmacotherapy in depression without comorbidity, at least in the long term. The same generalization seems to apply in the case of general anxiety disorder, with some nonpharmacological treatments, such as exposure techniques, more effective than others (Stein et al., 2005). Still, the research has the limitations already elaborated in chapter 2, and the findings may not easily apply to patients encountered in general psychotherapy practice since as a group these people have problems that may be distant from those involved in the RCTs reported, the gold standard for psychotherapy research (Roth & Fonagy, 2005; Westen et al., 2004). Further, the most efficacious nondynamic psychotherapies cited in the research literature are those classed under CBTs. However, relatively little good research has been done using other therapeutic modalities. The studies tend to be time limited and restricted by the criteria for the entity being studied.

Roth and Fonagy (2005), in their comprehensive, up-to-date volume, underscore the role that clinical judgment plays in the successful execution of therapeutic interventions, noting the place of a clear formulation of the patient's difficulties, including, as summarized by Millon (1996), the patient's mental attributes, beliefs, goals, and intentions. This formulation is necessarily complex and always evolving. Maruish (2002) is even clearer in articulating the components of an adequate case formulation (see also chapter 2).

In the end, distressingly, the rigorous clinician is left hanging. There is neither a general consensus nor adequate research to support the view that manualization—the use of manuals prescribing the steps for treating a particular entity—is reliably correlated with improved outcome, especially in real-world settings (Norcross et al., 2006). For one thing, treatment manuals are constructed from studies using RCTs, and the population of patients studied in these trials is restricted by the criteria for conducting the research from which the outcome data are derived. There is no definitive evidence that structured, empirically controlled therapies for specific entities such as depression (Roth & Fonagy, 2005) are more effective than those that are open ended and minimally structured. The intention to structure and make replicable what psychotherapists do is welcome in a field where accountability was previously almost nonexistent. However, attempting to entirely formularize a uniquely configured, sequentially evolving interpersonal intervention as complex and dynamic as psychotherapy is not even conceivable except under strictly controlled research conditions. Again, note that most of the available studies of psychotherapy were done using behavioral techniques, limiting the universality of the models for treatment derived. Finally, simply because a clinical phenomenon has been studied says nothing about the reliability of the studies. Many studies lack controls, are woefully limited in duration, lack adequate follow-up so that recurrences of the studied conditions are missed (Hass et al., 2002) and employ assessment measures that are too limited in scope to be clinically incisive.

Clinical judgment and other coveted nonspecific factors such as therapeutic alliance and congruence within the therapy relationship are not well enough standardized to be formally incorporated into these studies of therapeutic outcome. If one is to believe the recommendations of the Division 29 task force of the American Psychological Association, commissioned first in 1999 (Norcross, 2002), the therapy relationship makes the most significant contribution to psychotherapy outcome independent of the specific type of treatment. Efforts to promulgate general psychotherapy guidelines and ESTs without considering the central contribution of the therapy relationship therefore appear to be seriously incomplete and misleading. According to the Division 29 task force, the therapy relationship acts in concert with discrete interventions, and tailoring the therapy relationship to specific patient needs and characteristics enhances the effectiveness of the treatment (Addis, 1997; Norcross et al., 2006; see also American Psychological Association, 2002a).

The Challenge for Responsible Psychotherapists

How to carry out our duty to our patients when we are not certain about the factors that optimize psychotherapy? It is with this mission that Phil Erdberg and I originally undertook our project more than 15 years ago when we began our study of what we ultimately called the three-person therapy field. The designation "three-person therapy field" acknowledges the critical place that a psychologist-assessor plays in our work. He or she is not just another member of the treatment team but, rather, has an irreplaceable, permanent place in providing feedback about the patient's psychology and the developments, positive and negative, within the therapy. The psychologist-assessor is expected to respond to questions the therapist and patient submit before and after his or her formal psychological assessment, is called on regularly to reassess the patient, and is available for on-the-spot consultations at any time.

When we undertook this first project, we were well aware that definitive guidelines for selecting the optimal types and frequency of treatment for a particular patient or category of patient were not available. We recognized that practitioners made unsubstantiated claims about their ability to know what treatment requirements could most benefit a particular patient. We witnessed psychotherapies that went on inexorably without either patient or therapist questioning whether the patient was progressing, whether there was a better way to treat, when and whether treatment should stop, or even whether a treatment respite was in order when the patient asked for one.

Such was the state of the art when the Center was created by Diane Engelman and myself and the studies that led to its development were carried out. We recognized that we were flying blind then, and in many ways we still are. In fact, our basic position is that much is not known and may never be fully known about how effective psychotherapy works. Exactly what parameters to introduce to maximize a therapy's benefits with a particular patient and when to introduce each will probably always be elusive. In addition, requirements of a psychotherapy not only change over time but always consist of a mix of therapist and patient influence.

The result of this shifting and demanding set of conditions is to keep the treatment team on its toes. No method or methods of assessment, monitoring, and treatment are unequivocally reliable and ecologically valid, and certainly none is likely to continue to yield therapeutic benefit indefinitely. Some will be more effective than others, at least for a time. The clinical requirements of a psychotherapy are likely to seem less predictable than those framing a treatment in physical medicine, whether or not they really are. The implication for the Center is that we always expect surprises and posture ourselves accordingly. We are also clear about another conundrum. While we as medical practitioners need to take responsibility for our work and insist that it be demonstrably effective, often all we can know is when it is succeeding or failing, not precisely why. If we as psychotherapists are not ready to acknowledge our uncertainties by seeking consultation and, when needed, gracefully bowing out of the therapist's role, we are abusing our power and in effect betraying our sacred charge as therapists.

And so the plot thickens. As serious psychotherapists, we are faced with myriad choices. Do we emphasize the relationship over technique? To what extent should the collaborative feedback from the patient and psychologist-assessor be influential in structuring and modifying the plan for treatment? What about that which we do not know as we enter and move on in a psychotherapy? And what do we do about the subjectivity we as psychotherapists always encounter in our therapy work? In brief, how close can we come to realizing the ideal of replicable methods and demonstrated results, that is, the medical model for psychotherapy as described by Wampold (2001)? Of more pertinence is whether this is an ideal we should be aspiring toward, especially as we advocate and continue to evolve our own version of "evidence-based" diagnosis and treatment monitoring. Most likely, the answer is yes. After all, isn't "evidence based" a proper designation for the collaborative and assessment supported measures we are advocating?

CHAPTER FOUR

Our View

How often have you been confounded and amazed when the person you are working with suddenly sheds age-old problems and unwanted habits, excited as they discover heretofore unknown interests and capabilities? Making matters more interesting, these changes are likely to occur out of sync with deliberate, orchestrated measures to create these changes. My claim is that the real goal of psychotherapy is to reach the point where therapist and patient create this kind of magic together. Required is that the therapist finds an alive place to hook into the patient's personal world, joining in his creative process. Far less written about is the requirement that the patient needs also to tap the lifeblood of the therapist and equally facilitate the therapist's creative processes.

On any given day when I am with patients, I can tell when this mutual creativity is missing. On those days, I feel bored and get tired early, wondering what retirement might be like. Imagine!

My other three books (Frankel, 1995, 2000, 2007) are about the outlines of this largely nonverbal, intensely interpersonal process. There I formulate my view about how a psychotherapy patient is engaged to discover his or her latent treatment needs and unappreciated potential. I call the product of this effort "conjunction" and the progression through which it is reached the "conjunctive process." In *Hidden Faults* (2000), I focus on the place of disruptions in therapeutic rapport, that is, therapeutic disjunctions, resetting the frame from which the therapist and patient think and work so that a burst of creativity is possible for both. In *Making Psychotherapy Work* (2007),

I call a similar development from the therapist's side the "leap of inference." The precursor experience consists of feedback between therapist and patient that occurs as the two exchange the authority to know and lead in the therapy. Look closely at the events in a therapy, and you should be able to identify these shifts as they occur. Underpinning these exchanges and, for that matter, therapeutic movement altogether is a more subtle level of alternating and reciprocated communications I call "reciprocal knowing." Fully utilizing the potential that these deliberate and implicit operations provide requires the therapist to temporarily cease formulating within the therapy, a psychological maneuver I call "deliberate disorientation." It is here that the therapist allows him- or herself to become aware of the latent themes being played out by the two and the patient's unstated goals for the therapy, at times as they interdigitate with the therapist's (Chused, 1991; Frankel, 2007; Grotstein, 1981; Ogden, 1982, 1986; Schwaber, 1996).

In these books, I underscore the centrality of this complex, largely nonverbal communication. As a tribute to the power of this nonverbal exchange, discovery and personal change by the patient often lack coordination with purposeful therapeutic efforts to orchestrate this movement. Returning to chapter 3, this observation seems thoroughly compatible with the observations of Wampold (2001) and like-minded colleagues who report research findings, largely from meta-analyses, that affirm the centrality of nonspecific, contextual factors in psychotherapy efficacy. However, unlike me, they seem comfortable with the conclusion that specific factors, such as the choice of therapy technique, patient education, or socialization experience, pale next to the importance of nonspecific interpersonal factors. Apart from techniques that intentionally promote insight and perhaps behaviorally oriented symptom-focused approaches, they see limited distinction between these structured modes of intervention as they bear on therapeutic outcome.

In contrast with Wampold's position, my assumption when undertaking the project described in this book included my clinically based conviction that with the requisite nonspecific factors in place, specific factors may be quite relevant to therapeutic outcome. Like Wampold, others take the opposite position. Supporting their views are meta-analyses of the literature on psychotherapy dating from as early as 1980 (Smith, Glass, & Miller, 1980) showing effect sizes demonstrating that the therapist's training, theoretical orientation, and experience (summarized in Lambert, 2004) are relatively unimportant to therapy outcome.

I believe an analogy to antibiotics has at least some validity here. It would be poor medical practice to administer an antibiotic prior to doing a physical examination and without the appropriate bacterial or viral cultures.

What if the patient had a viral hepatitis and because of a sore throat and fever was treated for a bacterial infection? Worse yet, what if the sore throat and fever were the early symptoms of immune system failure, as in AIDS? How irrelevant can this analogy be when specific diagnostic tests and treatments are being developed at a breakneck pace to target the genetic and biochemical basis of psychiatric and neurological derangements and the field of psychiatry is moving ever closer to matching symptoms and syndromes to treatments?

Just 40 years ago, prominent psychiatrists were arguing that the central etiology of schizophrenia could be located in dysfunctional family patterns (Lidz, 1968). It may be worth remembering that one of the main proponents of this view was Theodore Lidz, for years chairman of the prestigious Department of Psychiatry at Yale. Having known him while I was in training, it is hard for me to think of his choice in taking this position as ideologically or politically motivated. In fact, at the time, he was considered to be a bit of a theoretical maverick, and his views about the family and its potential role in mental illness seemed refreshing to many of us. Also neglected then—and sometimes now—in diagnosis and treatment is acknowledgment of the ubiquity of trauma and the effect of preverbal experiences in creating adult psychiatric disturbance. Prominent psychiatrists and psychologists in those days argued that virtually all psychiatric disturbance was based on intrapsychic conflict, with some of them focusing on early loss and depravation as well (Mahler, 1972). Strange to remember how hopelessly isolated people—such as my good friend and hero Calvin Settlage (1992), who took the latter, developmental view about psychopathology—were made to feel by the classical psychoanalysts who tenaciously held to Freud's instinctual conflict theory.

So are Wampold and his colleagues wrong, even atavistic? Hardly. They are good, solid, contemporary researchers who know statistics cold. My claim is that they are simply missing the appropriate research data to draw firm conclusions about the place of specific factors in psychotherapy. Of course, like in most humanistic disciplines, there is a raging political debate that may be influencing their convictions. Sadly, as we consider the possibility of political contamination in current diagnosis and treatment, we probably should think of the Kingston Trio's song that began with "they're rioting in Africa" and concluded with "and I don't like anybody very much." That is, for whatever nonscientific reason, some groups of psychologists and psychiatrists have become hopelessly polarized for the moment, with the involved psychiatrists rabidly defending their medical model and psychologists tending to favor interpersonal therapeutic measures.

I actually do not suspect Wampold and colleagues of having political objectives in giving so much credit to contextual factors in making psychotherapy work. I personally find their conclusions remarkably freeing, and I believe that they are probably right as far as they go. Still, one cannot help but emerge from immersion in Wampold's writings without the feeling of having been in the middle of a polemical debate. Wampold's (2001) book, for example, seems to have an argumentative edge, and I believe that his chapters are too incomplete in what they cover to be fully convincing. Norcross's (2002) edited book is more complete but still thin in arguments for the possible value of specific techniques in psychotherapy, as, for example, they are codified in empirically supported treatment protocols.

More on My Method

Missing so far from the account I have given of my earlier writing is the place of our collaborative model of psychotherapy in identifying the most effective therapeutic approach for a particular case (Frankel, 2007). Earlier, I referred to this model of orchestrating psychotherapy as the conjunctive model (Frankel, 2007). First, nothing in psychotherapy takes place outside the context of intersubjectivity and mutual influence (Aron, 1996; Levenson, 1998; Mitchell, 1998; Slavin & Kriegman, 1998). Minimizing the impact of the therapist's needs and biases on this interpersonal operation would be to adulterate it hopelessly. The desired product of psychotherapy is an ever-evolving, shared conjunctive process leading to creative change, not just for the patient but for the therapist as well (Frankel, 2000, 2007).

Is this viewpoint—legitimizing the therapist's and not just the patient's benefits from participating in a treatment—a perversion of the psychotherapy process, a study in boundary violation? I hope not since my goal is not to deny the therapist credit for his or her hard-won technical expertise. Certainly, we choose our personal medical doctors after carefully taking into account their training and experience. It is no different for psychotherapists. But to imagine that a therapist has the corner on the truth or that his or her biases do not inform his or her choices is like pretending that your medical doctor will not be personally affected by your complaints and opinions or that you should not seek second opinions. In my mind, arguing that position would indiscriminately grant the therapist authority based on the myth of his or her omniscience.

Also central to my model of treatment is the place of collaboration in a fruitful psychotherapy. If the required part of psychotherapy is the conjunctive, contextual aspect and the added value is introduced by the decision about what specific measures are adopted by the two, the remaining question is how and when these procedures are decided on. My claim is that therapy decisions need to be guided by data, including data obtained clinically by an experienced practitioner and through psychological assessment as laid out in our diagnostic and monitoring procedures at the Center for Collaborative Psychology and Psychiatry. Also important, these data are the product of the therapist's and patient's shared appraisal of the patient's needs. The feedback loop between therapist and patient is continually directed at incorporating the always-changing nature of the patient's condition into the therapy sequence. The resulting plan for how to proceed in therapy exists in part on an intuitive level, sometimes shared and sometimes not. As these operations are consciously accessible to therapist and patient, they become the subject of their discussion. Note that in our model, we have included one additional loop in this circuit: that involving a psychologist-assessor.

The important point here is that one cannot know in advance which techniques, contextual or specific, will yield the best results in a psychotherapy. Unfortunately, this uncertainty creates a dilemma for the empirically supported treatment advocates among us. A set of rules about how to conduct a particular psychotherapy will, of necessity, become inaccurate or even misguided over time. Guidelines may work for a while, but the shared and individual subjectivities making up the therapy mandate that they will become less optimal over time. The described challenge to preestablished guidelines for conducting psychotherapy is exactly what confronted us as we began to develop protocols for assessment and monitoring of therapy progress at the Center. If cookbooks are of limited practical value in psychotherapy because of the latter's ever-shifting subjective substrate, how then to develop a set of therapeutic and assessment measures that enable a therapist to transcend the lack of accountability so common for conventional psychotherapy practice? As important, our diagnostic and monitoring guidelines would have to be cost effective and manageable enough in office-based practice that interested psychotherapists would actually embrace them. Added to the challenge is the requirement that the clinical techniques we recommend be straightforward enough that therapists other than ourselves would not only use them but welcome them as well.

I do not claim that we at the Center have mastered this problem. To provide clinically relevant data, we are tempted to rely on the psychological and neuropsychological assessments we have developed. In addition to completing the extensive initial testing battery every 18 months, we ask patients to agree to a much briefer reevaluation on a biannual basis. However, in our enthusiasm for our procedures, we know that we can underestimate the infinitely complex and discontinuous nature of the psychotherapy process, believing that we have found the optimal way to guide therapist and patient. Interestingly, we have come to fully believe in the value of the assessment and techniques we advocate at the Center. Are we wrong? Yes and no. Yes, the technique I arrived at for Gary, the patient described next, has worked well. No, in that the success to which I am referring may be short lived, and whether the technique is the optimal in any particular psychotherapy has to be resubstantiated each time.

So much for certainty and definitely for being overconfident. In fact, I believe our commitment to be tentative about our opinions is the formula for therapeutic success. Its essence seems to be our willingness to "not know." Our thinking this way seems critical if patients are to develop faith in us. Of course, some patients want us to be absolutely sure of ourselves, to lay out just what they should do to reach their goals. Our experience is that these are the people who are least likely to be able to fully participate in therapy work. They often require the therapist to think for them and are limited in their ability to self-reflect. On the extreme end of this group, qualifying for the diagnosis of borderline personality disorder, are patients like Gary, described in the next section (Linehan 1993).

I believe that our emphasis on collaboration between the therapist, patient, and psychologist-assessor ensures that the essence of the psychotherapy, the critical "contextual" factors that Wampold (2001) names, is being preserved. Still, we are not so certain that specific interventions pale in importance as compared to those that are the less deliberately orchestrated and contextual. To guide us, however, our model goes one major step further than theirs by always incorporating formal measures to ensure the therapist and patient that their diagnosis remains reasonably on target and that adequate progress is occurring.

How We Do It

The Impossible Patient: Gary

At 47, Gary was going nowhere. The situation, by anyone's standards, was simply hideous. Gary had been to one of the finest men's colleges. To boot, he was admitted a year early at age 16 without graduating from high school. He simply decided one day to apply, and presto, he was admitted.

That was in the early days. Now he was misanthropic to a fault, fighting with everyone who crossed his path. It wasn't that they simply offended him; in his view, they meant to offend him.

And, of course, that's where I came in. Whatever I said sent Gary into a rage. What did I mean when I said that his friend George couldn't paint as well as Gary? How presumptuous of me. Worse, when I didn't echo his own ideas about people's motivations, he felt offended and pouted for the rest of the day. It may be worth noting that his parents had given up. They had joined an organization for people with borderline children, wished Gary would consider Linehan's dialectal-behavioral therapy treatment, and had long ago decided that Gary would never achieve anything of value to society. He would always be too depressed to work and too socially isolated to make friends. He would never marry. He insisted that he was an artist but had never sold anything in spite of his numerous "completed" works of art.

So what was "broke" here? The easy answer is, everything. Not only was Gary larger and more clumsy than anyone else I knew, but his psychological development had been thoroughly stunted as well. And, worse, Gary was one of the most unappealing human beings I'd ever met: argumentative, arrogant, not self-reflective.

How do you fix the whole human being, especially when they are more than old enough to be a finished product? At least that was the essence of what I found myself asking about my work with Gary. Oddly, it was Gary who provided the answer: "Use traditional therapeutic technique so I can't confuse what you are saying for some quirky personal agenda of yours. Also, I want to get to know and work cooperatively with my parents again, in spite of all the damage I believed they have done to me. I'd like you to arrange at least one meeting with them."

Perhaps because it began to make some sense or maybe because I found myself on the edge of exhaustion, I slowly began to consider Gary's request. Gary's allegation was that his father had been depressed and abusive from Gary's early childhood. Gary claimed that he, Gary, had been traumatized at that time, losing all confidence in his own worth and future in spite of his impressive academic achievements. It seemed logical that Gary could be reenacting this kind of trauma with me in the therapy. A red light was flashing, however. What better way to create confusion in someone given to projection than to cross their adult boundaries, as he was inviting me to do if I agreed to meet with his parents? Doing so was also risky considering Gary's general intolerance for almost anything I said and did. As an individual psychotherapy maneuver, it certainly was unusual given Gary's age. Nonetheless, meeting with Gary's parents, either with or separate from Gary, seemed like a logical next therapeutic measure.

I held out for several weeks, but finally I was so worn out that I yielded.

From that point, holding our trajectory was neither smooth nor easy. The first step was to contain and confront Gary's usual seething rage at me. In fact, I have never felt as reviled in my 35 years as a psychiatrist as I did then by Gary. He not only didn't like me—he hated me. While my meeting with his parents was his idea, once I started to do so, he repeatedly threatened to sue me because of my alleged breaches of his confidentiality. He called a psychiatrist friend of mine, also a friend of his family, and itemized my infractions of proper psychotherapeutic technique. He began to come late for sessions, sometimes he failed to show up, and his sessions were so saturated with his angry withholding that I could hardly wait until each one was over.

Technically, the problem for Gary and the key to our success as I formulated it was that, while Gary's demand was that I resign as his therapist, his parents would not hear of it. There had been too many psychotherapists, and this time he had to see it through, or they would simply cut him off financially. The next step would be for him to go on welfare and move to public housing. See it through, or else.

I agreed with Gary's parents and resolved within myself to carry on with the therapy regardless of how technically and emotionally hard it became. I told both Gary and his parents about my decision. I had in mind that this choice would ensure the continuity of the treatment. It would work a bit like the martial arts strategy of trapping an opponent by taking advantage of his or her own momentum. In this case, that momentum was Gary's implicit intention to remain an emotional cripple and financially dependent.

At the same time, I did what I was told by Gary and labored to make the changes in my therapy technique he insisted on. Also, since I had never been convinced that he was as disturbed as he and everyone else believed and in particular since I did not think he was bipolar or had the obscure developmental disorder his previous therapist described, I suggested neuropsychological testing and a neurological work-up. Weakly, he agreed that he too really wanted to know more about what was wrong with him. Nonetheless, characteristically, the promise for his future that the planned assessments held were never acknowledged by Gary. He continued to be as insulting and grumpy with me as ever. But he was cooperative with the work-up and apparently looked forward to the clarification it might provide.

Wanting this intervention to be as powerful as possible, I privately orchestrated a meeting between Gary, the neurologist and neuropsychologist who tested him, and myself. Prior to this meeting, I learned that, as I suspected, the MRI of Gary's brain was normal, and so was a subsequent PET scan of his brain. The neuropsychological testing showed no evidence of severe psychopathology, save the emotional instability of Gary's borderline personality disorder and long-standing unsociable habits. Once I learned about these findings, I asked the neurologist and neuropsychologist to be clear and confrontational in our meeting with Gary, as much as possible forcing him to hear testimony about his heretofore underestimated assets.

No doubt, there was plenty of work left for us. We had Gary's view of himself as a lifelong patient, his counterproductive habits, and his exquisite sensitivity to rejection to manage and reverse. He had long ago scuttled the idea of developing a career, and that goal had to be revived. Also, Gary's medications needed to be reduced so that he could begin to think clearly and concentrate.

Thankfully, Gary's anticipated negative response to the good news was short lived. Since being informed at age 47 that his being normal could signal that he would be required to behave normally and even work, Gary might have been expected to rebel and develop new problems or simply not accept or even hear what he was told. In contrast, Gary slowly became more optimistic. Within a few months, he stopped demanding that I bow out and even asked to see the vocational counselor I had earlier recommended. He also took the first steps toward entering a dialectical behavior therapy group. He began to warm up to his parents. In our sessions, the misanthrope began to be easier to be with.

In chapter 5, I describe our treatment model. As I hope I have conveyed in the discussion of my work with Gary, we are guided by three simple but never easy-to-achieve principles: determine what is broken about the patient, devise a scheme for fixing it, and then do whatever the fix requires. Standing on theoretical ceremony is out of the question. So much of what is taught and done as psychotherapy emphasizes form rather than substance. We know the rules, but we also know that connecting usefully with human beings requires infinite flexibility. Psychotherapy, if it is to be a process in which two human beings meaningfully understand each other and connect, requires ingenuity. The product is a personal and indeed an interpersonal reevaluation, a transformative process I call creative change. In the best circumstances, the patient and therapist are deeply affected in this process, and both emerge changed (Frankel, 2000).

I was the first one in his life to take Gary's claim that he had been traumatized as a child seriously. He said he had hardly trusted anyone afterward, always running from his parents and all the others who he believed were out to take advantage of and humiliate him. Accepting the veracity of Gary's claims and finding a way to make his life more tolerable were keys to the required fix. Expectations of normalcy were put in place. The antipsychotic medication that his previous psychiatrists had prescribed and that he insisted he needed were reduced or eliminated from the long list of drugs he was taking. Friends like George slowly and noisily came to be seen as more trustworthy, and Gary even reconciled with his parents. This was the fix, and its result was reassuring.

Gary's attitude toward treatment began to shift. Apparently during this period, he had also decided that this time therapy was going to work. Using a progressively interactive version of the psychotherapy method that he so judiciously insisted on, during the next 2-year period of meeting twice weekly, we did what we could to plumb the deepest recesses of his trauma and to begin to reclaim Gary's long-buried self. In parallel, he became more cooperative and introspective. He also began to be attractive, even a bit handsome, as he decided it was now safe to pursue a relationship with a woman.

Of course, the path was full of bumps and traps. It was not unusual, at least in the beginning, to receive a call from an apparently half-dead Gary telling me that he didn't have a friend in the world or accusing me of violating his trust through improper therapy technique. He continued to quit treatment periodically, always returning restored in a week or two.

By now, you may be able to guess the next step. Gary's father, relieved, finally was able to come forward. He asked to meet with me to explore what kind of damage he might have done to Gary during his childhood and adolescence. He suspected that his own depressions and rages during Gary's childhood were instrumental in creating Gary's problems. He corroborated everything Gary told me: tantrums, beatings, and threats to abandon his children. His grand admission was that he probably should never have gotten married and agreed to have children given his state of mind during that time. After all, his own father had abandoned him for 10 years from ages 5 through 15, going to a distant city and living with relatives.

Oh, and I was fixed as well. Being relieved of feelings that were close to repulsion for one's patient is a remarkable gift.

Not yet addressed is the magic—how it really worked between Gary and me.

At first, Gary distrusted and even hated me. To be honest, I felt similarly about him. At the end of each tormenting session, I wanted to chuck the whole thing. I told my wife privately that Gary was the most difficult patient I had ever treated. In consultation with colleagues, I was advised to give up the work with Gary or get tough, setting clear boundaries on Gary's abuse of me and expecting that he take the work seriously and be a contributing partner in our therapy. Actually, when I tried to insist that he commit himself to doing his part, he became enraged. "I don't have to do anything I don't want to do. The only person in here with responsibilities is you. You are simply supposed to keep your mouth shut and do therapy." When I then tried to draw the line and told him that his "attitude felt abusive to me," he simply asked for the name of another therapist and resolved to quit treatment.

In fact, Gary's only acknowledged reason for staying in therapy with me at that point was that his parents made it mandatory. They were paying for the treatment and insisted that he had made impressive progress with me and that our work proved that previous therapy attempts had been a waste of their money. In response to my encouragement, they made it clear to Gary that if he did not attempt to work out his problems with me, they would cut off his funding. Years before, they had witnessed my treatment of friends' adolescent children and said that they had been impressed by the risks I was willing to take and by the outcome of these therapies. Each of these patients had been in treatment previously and had failed to make substantial gains.

From his viewpoint, why did Gary stay in treatment with me through those insufferably difficult months? One possibility is that Gary was actually relieved by his parents' insistence that he stay in treatment and work his problems through, as long as he did not have to take overt responsibility for that decision. Supporting this speculation is the observation that teenagers often put their welfare in their parents' hands and then act as if they bear no responsibility for the decisions the parents are forced to make. In fact, adolescence was the stage of development that Gary had apparently bypassed, electing instead not to give up his idyllic preadolescent sense that he would be taken care of forever. Conscious disavowal of needs and demands is typical of teenagers. The adolescent forces his parents to take responsibility for his welfare while acting as if he has no place in their decisions. The result is that the teenager creates the illusion for himself that he is competently controlling his own life while privately ensuring that his parents will be protective no matter how outrageous his behavior becomes. Using this mechanism, Gary, his own complicity implied, was forced to do what he had never done: work things through when they got tough.

And what about my reason for hanging in? After all, Gary did nothing but agitate me every time I saw him. I wonder why I did not fire him or at least capitalize on his threat to quit treatment. The best answer I can come up with is that I was impressed by Gary's imagination. I found it hard to believe that anyone with so much creative potential, anyone who could be as attractive as Gary when he was at his best, could be as crazy and intentionally hateful as he seemed when he was in one of his typical dismissive moods with me. Quite frankly, before we explored his early history, I never considered his problems to be related to early and repeated trauma in spite of my knowledge of how frequent trauma is retrospectively identified in the lives of adult borderline patients. My omission in part probably also reflected my distaste, even repulsion, for his identity as a psychological cripple and my intuition that this view of himself, while believed by everyone including Gary, was significantly contrived. Also, I knew enough about Gary's parents' current caretaking of Gary that I respected them and believed that Gary was falsely demonizing them.

What seemed like magic—keeping us together through thick and thin and eventually leading to our mutual transformation to trusting and believing in one another—was indeed just that: a kind of therapeutic magic. Hidden in the background and well disguised, I infer, was the admiration we felt for one another. In fact, I believe, neither of us wanted to give up. We both needed the breaks Gary frequently forced in our work. The timing of these may have actually been precise, with neither of us the least bit convinced of their possible therapeutic value at the time they occurred. Call it what you like: luck that Gary's parents knew enough about me to have blind faith in the possibility that I might be the one to finally help their son or relief that Gary experienced as he relinquished the hostile symbiotic-like tie with his parents, it nonetheless worked. In fact, it has worked so well that Gary remains devoted to our psychotherapy. At this point, he is enjoying a much improved personal life and a decent relationship with his parents and two previously estranged sisters, and I am still simply rubbing my eyes.

Common Factors in the Experience of Therapeutic Magic

The most convincing evidence that a treatment is working is, of course, its outcome. It is hard to argue with therapeutic success, especially if it is consistent with psychological and neuropsychological testing and follow-up.

While usually regarded as an inadequate source of reliable data in physical medicine and the hard sciences, critical evidence here also comes appreciably from the patient's personal testimony. I don't like being in this position. I would rather stick exclusively to the results of our Center's testing procedure in orchestrating and evaluating our work. But often I have no choice but to lean on these subjective reports. In addition, I would be deceiving myself if I minimized the fact that my strategy with Gary did not come about significantly as a result of my clinical judgment.

There is nothing faulty about this position as far as it goes. First, Gary would not submit to our testing procedure during our early months of work, and insisting that he do so would have been met with a raging "you're trying to control me." While in this frame of mind, Gary could hardly have been expected to undertake any kind of formal assessment. The result: no baseline measurement. Second, it is hard to imagine that during our painful struggle any assessment instruments, except possibly the Rorschach, would have provided evidence of the subtle progress we were apparently making. Third, other, nontangible factors are at work to make therapy succeed. For example, Gary's parents were sold on the value of the therapy with me. Their financial support made it possible for me to persist with Gary during his rages and threats to quit treatment. It was also important to me that other involved human beings confirmed the value of the therapy. Underscored here is the place of others in supporting psychotherapy, an interpersonal factor that is often only marginally credited as important in treatment, whether psychological or medical.

Success with Gary was elusive. For him to trust that I truly understood his experience, I apparently had to be battered in a way reminiscent of the abuse he experienced during his own childhood. However, that I could withstand such mistreatment and still remain committed to him and even that he might have something to say that interested me were equally important for him. Apparently, as he approached his 50th birthday, he needed someone to acknowledge how badly he had been mishandled as a child (this function is called "witnessing" by Auerhahn and Peskin, 2003). He was acutely aware that as the only male child, he had been chosen to replicate his father's own history of abuse and abandonment. He expected nothing less than a replay of his earlier battering experiences if he let his guard down with me as well. His belligerence had the partial purpose of attacking me in hope of diverting me from doing the same to him.

Notice the place of my own conversion in this process. I began by not believing that Gary could possibly have a point and was simply given to blaming others, a characteristic of borderline personality–disordered people in general. What we came up with was a willing participant-witness in his father, who confessed all. From there, self-reflection, searching for his own contribution to his difficulties, became less devastating for Gary, and he could become a productive partner in our work.

Of course, this development was not the end of our ordeal. In many ways, Linehan's writing (1993) predicts that Gary would continue his erratic and abusive behavior. Nonetheless, Gary finally became a reasonably willing partner in our psychotherapy. The next step was to invoke an appropriate albeit sometimes painful management strategy involving expectations and shared planning. Of course, my work with his parents, dissuading them from believing that Gary was terminally impaired and from continuing to unconditionally support him, was essential in achieving this aim. Although while Gary at first resisted undertaking the privileges and responsibilities of a 47-year-old, he silently began to think about finding an occupation and giving up his monthly allowance. This shift was Gary's doing, although he often still regularly blamed me for making it necessary.

And the reward? Slowly it dawned on Gary that he could now expect to begin a normal life and even to have the relationship and sexual experiences he claimed to crave.

A Word About Therapeutic Magic

What seems like magic—forcing remarkable change in both patient and therapist—is, of course, ultimately explicable. The key to understanding it is in noticing the gut-wrenching process around which it generates. Neither therapist nor patient escapes this ultimately constructive ordeal. Of course, at times patient and therapist work together seamlessly. However, it is worth asking whether the rewards from that kind of experience are as rich as when the therapist and patient are forced to recognize and face their essential differences. In *Hidden Faults* (Frankel, 2000), where I discuss therapeutic disjunctions, I distinguish between two types of disjunctions. In one, conjunctive disjunctions, there is simply a difference of opinion, and the problem is thoughtfully resolved. In the second type, typified by my rocky experience with Gary, a positive outcome is anything but guaranteed.

This second disjunctive process requires one or both therapeutic partners to come to terms with a position that seems disruptive to both of them. Ordinarily, the impact of this new reality is jolting and is forcefully resisted by one or both partners. From there, fur begins to fly. The patient feels that the therapist is unreasonable, and the therapist may feel desperate to find a way to make his or her point. For a long period, nobody is quite sure who is right. Or, worse, both are sure they are right. Working out of this dilemma is never easy. Yet it is almost always personally transforming for one or both partners.

In the very beginning of our work, I, like all his other therapists, thought Gary was crazy. Now most every meeting with him becomes delightful at some point. The change, which most certainly has occurred in both of us, is remarkable, me finding Gary credible, even wise, and Gary beginning to lead a productive life. This process, creative change (Frankel, 2000), is the guts of the conjunctive process I describe in *Making Psychotherapy Work* (Frankel, 2007).

The Next Chapter

It is time for me to describe the procedures we have evolved at the Center. To this point, I have surveyed the rationale for our adopting these assessment and monitoring techniques. Most important to the intention of this book is that our methods be useful clinically, be convenient, and be affordable enough for any psychotherapist to use in the office. They also need to be clearly enough articulated to be easily understood and applied by office-based psychotherapists. Said in another way, these procedures need to be publicly replicable. After all, therapeutic treatment is rarely practiced in a research setting, and the majority of those who are likely to use the Center's procedures described in chapter 5 are office based.

CHAPTER FIVE

Our Method and Procedures: Adults

In this chapter, I describe the procedures we use for assessment and treatment of adult patients at the Center for Collaborative Psychology and Psychiatry. Included are our assessment protocols, treatment guidelines, treatment monitoring procedures, and method of posttreatment follow-up. Of course, every one of our interventions is tailor-made for the individual patient and for each therapist–patient combination. Our technique allows, in fact requires, the two to regularly review and modify this assessment and treatment sequence to ensure that the treatment gets off to a good start. Exactly when the assessment should take place relative to the patient's initial contact with the therapist and when each reassessment should occur are matters of clinical judgment. The same principle applies in decisions about which tests and questionnaires to use, add, and subtract from our basic assessment protocol. This very flexibility and our insistence that clinical judgment play a central role in our decisions clearly distinguishes our work from that intended primarily for research.

While we want to contribute to the psychotherapy research literature, we cannot escape the fact that our patients are drawn from a typical clinical practice. They are ordinary people seeking help for their real problems, not for a neatly circumscribed set of symptoms. Generally, when working with this population, the problems encountered are multifaceted and incorporate a mixture of symptoms and personality deformations (Millon, 1996). Added are the psychological residua of past traumas and arrests in development that restrict the patient's capacity to relate fully and comfortably with others. As if this level of complexity weren't enough, there are also current stresses compromising the patient's emotional resources. These difficulties may be offset by the patient's unique strengths and configured by his or her cultural background.

Already you have a very complicated, essentially unclean picture. In brief, while the procedures we use must be validated (Chambless & Hollon, 1998, 2002; Chambless & Ollendick, 2001; Chambless et al. 1996), they also have to be effective. Their worth needs to be anchored in the patient's practical reality, demonstrated through improvements in the quality of his or her life (Westen, Novotny, & Thompson-Brenner, 2004).

Our methods are outlined here. None are applied religiously. If they were, it would compromise our flexibility, our capacity to modify our approach according to clinical requirements. Ideally, formal Center assessment and monitoring procedures come into play at set points in treatment. However, as will be discussed, in office-based practice it is often difficult or clinically injudicious to stick to such a schedule (Lamporpoulos et al., 2002). That said, the ideal sequence is as follows: initial meetings for the purpose of making a clinical assessment, psychological and neuropsychological testing by a psychologist-assessor, the creation and discussion of a plan of action that may or may not involve psychotherapy, and referral as appropriate. The evaluation is followed by the psychotherapy itself: its beginning, middle, and concluding phases. This entire operation is sustained by patient–therapist collaboration as well as an ongoing dialogue with the psychologist-assessor. Together with formal goal setting, resetting, and repeat testing, these operations form the technical basis of our method of assessment, treatment, and treatment monitoring.

Following the initial assessment and formulation of a tentative treatment plan, testing begins. Just prior to testing, the therapist and patient submit a set of questions and observations to be addressed by the psychologist-assessor. When the test data are in, a definitive treatment plan can be formulated, and psychotherapy can begin in earnest. As treatment progresses, the relatively objective test data are synthesized with the more subjective observations of the therapist, patient, and psychologist-assessor. Collaboration between all three keeps the therapist and patient on track, continually revising their understanding of one another's thinking and the direction of the therapy. It also creates an atmosphere within which the patient is likely to feel heard and able to advocate for him- or herself.

Of note is that keeping the therapist engaged should be as much a concern for therapy as maintaining the patient's interest and involvement. Although less is written about it, the patient has a constant, unofficial role in fueling the therapist's enthusiasm by being committed to the treatment and actively participating in creating the insight and change they seek.

The same principles apply in physical medicine. When the patient and even family fail to do their parts to sustain treatment, emotional and technical leverage are lost (Greenfield & Kaplan, 1985). The result is often lower satisfaction, adherence, and poorer biological and functional outcomes. By the same token, a decline in the physician's personal involvement in a treatment easily leads to a sterile process in which medical test results are followed in a reflexive manner, leading progressively to a decline in the patient's involvement (Duffy & Gordon, 2004; Frankel, Quill, & McDaniel, 2003; Lipkin, Putnam, & Lazare, 1995).

In short, the importance of collaborative truing mechanisms in therapeutic work, whether the treatment is medical or psychosocial, cannot be overstated. Involved are the patient, therapist or medical doctor, and, in our case, a psychologist-assessor. Family members may also be included directly or in the background.

Our Procedure for Assessment of Adults and for Monitoring Their Progress

Phase 1: The Initial Clinical Assessment

Overview

The goal of the initial assessment is to identify and begin to address the patient's manifest concerns. Over time, the patient's more subtle difficulties will be brought into focus, provided that the therapy work is carried out skillfully. The challenge at this point is to give the patient and therapist the opportunity to begin to get to know one another and for the patient to establish enough trust in the therapist to carry on with the evaluation. Especially during this initial phase, the patient's or, in the case of a child or an adolescent, the family's interest and willingness to cooperate can never be taken for granted.

The technical task at this point is to foster the getting-acquainted process while gathering as much pertinent current and past history about the patient's difficulties as possible, including relevant information from outside informants such as doctors and family members. Note that successfully constructing a picture of the patient's public and private life and background requires the patient to be forthcoming, often about information he or she is reluctant to reveal. That is, amassing the most complete and relevant history is an interpersonal as well as a technical challenge.

At the conclusion of this phase, the patient needs to be fully informed about and in agreement with Center procedures, including our initial and ongoing testing protocol. He or she also needs to be comfortable with the projected cost of the work. It is important in setting fees for the patient to realize that the commitment is one that needs to be sustained for the work to yield results. Not final at this point is the selection of treatment type. The patient will need to know of the many possible types of treatment and the potential benefits of each. He or she will probably also want to know the projected length of the assessment and treatment. He or she should be clear about our collaborative-consultative method and what it entails, including his or her part in sustaining it.

In clinical reality, a treatment approach can never be fixed. It needs to be reevaluated and modified in accordance with life events and treatment-based developments. Not the least of these influential factors, determining the course of treatment, are the therapist's personal contributions, including his or her evolving feelings about the patient (Frankel, 2000, 2007). There is no way to accurately judge these confounding influences as they bear on the pace and success of treatment. Considering the plethora of factors determining the course of a psychotherapy or a medical treatment, pity the poor patient whose medical doctor or psychotherapist sticks to a rigid treatment protocol, relinquishing the good judgment he or she brings as a result of his or her experience and intuition.

Case Example: Doreen

At age 49, Doreen, a single gay woman, seemed to be doing pretty well in her life. She had a thriving antique business. She began to collect and then sell antiques during her service in the Peace Corps, where she held important administrative positions from ages 21 through 30. She graduated from an excellent university and had plenty of friends, especially in other countries.

But Doreen wasn't happy.

For years, she neatly hid this disaffection, bolstering her mood with mind-altering drugs and assuaging her failing sense of vitality with travel and work in other countries. Unfortunately, the relief that substances provided came back to haunt her, and just prior to being referred to me, Doreen was diagnosed with a kidney condition brought on by her use of recreational drugs. Her unreflective lifestyle had suddenly evolved into a medical and, indeed, a psychiatric emergency.

The fact that I am not gay did not seem to trouble Doreen. While she was thoroughly acculturated into the gay community, she preferred relating to men and women who were comfortable with their sexual preference.

Entering into a productive psychotherapy, however, was not so easy for Doreen. First, she knew she might have to stop using drugs and so at first did not want to reveal to me how much and how often she used them. Her most pressing goal was to find a partner who was caring and stable. Her former partner had died in a motorcycle accident 3 years previously, and, worse, a year before her death, she ran off with another woman. Doreen turned to promiscuity and increased her use of drugs to drown out her despair.

Doreen realized that she was handicapped by the lack of an early model for committed relationship. Her mother and father were divorced when she was 6, after years of intolerable discord. Her brother was depressed and eventually committed suicide. The ultimate decision during her stint in the Peace Corps to shift her geographical center to the Middle East was admittedly Doreen's way of getting away from the nightmarish family environment that persisted even after her parents' divorce.

Returning to Center procedure, I met with Doreen six times, three or four more than are usual at the onset of a typical Center evaluation. We continued with preliminary visits until she lowered her guard enough to commit to a full work-up and give me what I thought was an accurate report of her current problems. Patient caution and ambivalence often requires us to modify the time frame and even structure of our initial evaluation. We are then faced with the challenge of sustaining the thoroughness of the work-up while making the necessary concessions to maintain the patient's full commitment. As illustrated by Doreen, one consequence of these revised requirements may be that the work-up will be prolonged. At other times, more optional parts of the work-up, such as more extensive components of neuropsychological testing, may need to be postponed or even eliminated.

A Detailed Account of the Initial Assessment

The initial clinical assessment is conducted by a Center-trained therapist and usually requires a meeting devoted exclusively to taking a history, a review of records, and two to four clinical meetings, each of which includes at least some formal history taking.

In addition to the history recorded by the therapist, the patient is asked to fill out data sheets for gathering information about his or her current life. Contacts are made with other mental health professionals who have treated the patient and, when relevant, with key family members. The patient, and in the case of a child or an adolescent, parents and teachers as well will also be asked to complete history and symptom checklists. Having the patient record background material, including a clinical history, cuts short the contact time required for this part of the assessment process.

Home and school visits may be arranged for children or adolescents and are described in chapter 6.

Do note that the final harvesting of historical material may take months. Some of the forms given to our patients are extensive, and people often do not like to fill out forms, especially long ones. The resulting delay in completing all parts of the evaluation is another example of an unavoidable departure from the ideal. Nonetheless, the information being solicited is crucially important to the work undertaken. Also, the use of questionnaires can result in enormous savings in time and cost since it reduces the face-to-face contact required to get essential background information.

At the conclusion of the initial assessment, the therapist arrives at a preliminary case formulation with a tentative diagnostic impression involving personality, psychosocial, and biological factors; works it over with the patient; and commits it to writing. The therapist identifies data still to be collected as well as other assessments, such as educational or medical, that are needed or desired. The patient's ability to afford treatment as well as his or her support systems should be factored prominently into the assessment and incorporated into the recommendations.

Plans for the testing may have to be postponed until the patient understands its purpose and accepts its value. In fact, it was necessary to wait until Doreen had been in treatment with me for 4 months before she could seriously consider testing. Like so many other patients, she first needed to assure herself that I was capable of appreciating the emotional gravity of her needs before she agreed to go further. The actual testing did not start until 6 months after our work started. The final determination of length and frequency of visits and an approximation of the likely duration of treatment is delayed until the first testing battery is completed.

See appendix A at the end of this chapter for more detail about this part of the evaluation process.

Phase 2: Testing, Feedback, and Formulation of a Treatment Plan

It is hoped that, by this point, several weeks and usually no more than 3 months into the assessment, the patient will have arrived at his initial impressions of the therapist and therapy and be able to make a commitment to the full assessment. The therapist needs to be satisfied that the patient's expectations for the treatment are workable as well. At the end of the assessment, the diagnosis, treatment plan, and predictions from this phase should be committed to writing by the therapist and reviewed collaboratively with the patient.

This phase also must be broached for the patient and therapist to formulate testing questions for the psychologist-assessor. The questions should be recorded. This document should also contain separate statements from the therapist and patient identifying the patient's key problems and any other information that might help guide the psychologist-assessor. The patient is also encouraged to remark about his or her therapy experience to date and especially issues about which he or she is unsettled. Often the commentary that the patient provides is surprising to the therapist, tipping him or her off to trouble before it infects the therapy work.

A convenient way for both therapist and patient to record and follow issues as they evolve in treatment is by frequently, ideally biweekly or monthly, completing the Target Complaint and Goal Attainment questionnaires. These self-report questionnaires are brief. They are simple devices (check sheets) for organizing and recording the patient's and the therapist's concerns and goals for psychotherapy. The magnitude of Doreen's anxiety, for example, was not always obvious to me as we talked. She was, however, quite clear about it in her responses to these questionnaires.

With the completion of testing, at the end of this part of the assessment, the psychologist-assessor can determine which test parameters and clinical markers should be most closely monitored in the treatment. These may change as the patient's personal requirements and the focus of the treatment shift.

Note that the collaborative testing (Finn & Fischer, 1997; Fischer, 2000) and treatment model we use (Frankel, 2007) is predicated on the recognition that new past and current personal data will continue to emerge as they become relevant and accessible. In part, the patient's report of manifest problems gives way to latent, previously hidden or inaccessible complaints and life problems as well as the discovery of unappreciated sources of strength, talents, and support systems. In fact, the emergence and consolidation of these data will frequently parallel the synthetic aspects of the therapy work itself.

A Comment About Testing

There are innumerable psychological and neuropsychological tests available for the purpose of making a diagnostic assessment and monitoring change in a psychotherapy. According to Meyer et al.'s (2001) extensive meta-analytic review, this testing often proves to be as dependable as medical tests. However, to be useful for psychosocial treatment, the findings require integration with descriptive information about the patient. Further, the human factor again enters when these data are communicated and used according to the assessor's and the therapist's clinical judgment. It is worth noting that, as in physical medicine, psychological or neuropsychological test data are most reliable when matched with similar data from several sources.

Widely used psychological assessment instruments include the following:

1. Problem-solving tests, such as the Rorschach, and projective tests, such as the Thematic Apperception Test (TAT). These instruments provide data about a patient's inner world and require a great deal of time to score, although the Rorschach does have a computer-scoring utility of some value.
2. Traditional personality assessments, such as the Minnesota Multiphasic Personality Inventory and Personality Assessment Inventory (PAI). These instruments can be entirely computer scored and are accompanied by a report that can be generated easily.
3. Self-report screens, including the Symptom Checklist-90 (SCL-90) and the Outcome Questionnaire-45, both symptom-oriented questionnaires, and others, including the Beck and Hamilton Depression and Anxiety Scales, which assess specific problem areas. These screens have been normed using large populations, and, while limited in the information they provide, can be clinically useful.
4. Less popular, subjectively focused assessment batteries, such as the Adult Attachment Projective, the Inventory of Interpersonal Problems, the Roberts Apperception Test for children and adolescents, and the Scale of Psychological Capacities. The Scale of Psychological Capacities is more cumbersome than the others since it requires a person separate from the therapist to administer and rate the findings.
5. Briefer self-report questionnaires, such as the Goal Attainment Scale and the Target Complaint Inventory, that aid in tracking a patient's clinical status.

In this list, I have named only a handful of the available assessment instruments.

The Center's assessment and monitoring procedure has been created with this entire range of assessments in mind. In selecting which tests to use and at what frequency, reliability, clinical usefulness, ease of administration, and affordability have been the determining factors.

Doreen Continued

Testing underscored Doreen's high level of anxiety and tendency to experience apprehension in the form of physical symptoms. One of her early complaints was that she was not able to focus during sex. Most of these complaints proved medically baseless, simply a manifestation of worry. But worry about what? Not obvious at first, probably because of her strikingly feminine appearance, was the fact that through repeated disappointments and originally because of recognizing the difference between her sexual preferences and those of most other girls during her teens, Doreen had become convinced that she was physically and personally unattractive. She carried this insecurity into each new relationship, certain that she would ultimately be judged unappealing. She was always shocked whenever she received a compliment from a partner.

Then there was Doreen's neediness. At one point, she so desperately wanted a steady partner that she deceived herself into believing that a particularly obliging woman who showed interest in her, Bobbie, would be perfect as a life partner. Of interest is that, unlike Doreen, Bobbie did not have a college education and worked as a low-level corporate employee. Within weeks, Bobbie, with Doreen's encouragement, moved into Doreen's lovely home and soon had Doreen straightening out the disarray in her financial affairs. Providing these services for Bobbie required not only Doreen's time but also her money.

Fortunately for our work, Doreen was a good historian. She dutifully filled out the Center's history forms. This information strongly suggested that the background for Doreen's vulnerability included a needy and punitive father who left his family for as long as a week at a time whenever he was angry at Doreen's mother or his children. Doreen's high-powered but quixotic mother was of little help in these situations, which she handled by simply shrugging them off. Her younger brother was a mess, attempting suicide twice during his teens. To survive emotionally, Doreen was forced to care for her father with the kind of exquisite attentiveness she later wanted from lovers and now was showering on Bobbie. No questions asked. For the record, her father's neediness and self-centered obtuseness was frighteningly close to Bobbie's exploitative behavior.

The information I have just conveyed is a product of the early clinical hours, the testing questions Doreen formulated, her history, and, finally, the psychological-neuropsychological testing itself. I used this information in at least two ways. I wove it, as well as my clinical observations, into a case formulation, and I made some initial probes of Doreen's ability to use the insights derived, which seemed promising. After some exploration, I told Doreen that the nature and actual basis of her anxiety and somatization were mysterious to me but that we would work hard to understand them. I also began the process of weaning her off all substances.

See appendices A and B at the end of this chapter for more detail about the Center's clinical assessment and testing.

Phase 3: Treatment

This phase unfolds over time. Formal assessments of therapy progress occur approximately once every 6 months. A record of the patient's current problems and therapy goals is kept in the therapist's notes and through the patient and therapist completing the Target Complaint and Goal Attainment Scales on a biweekly or monthly basis.

Complexity enters the therapy field as the therapist and patient inevitably develop divergent impressions of therapy requirements and of each other (Frankel, 2007). In *Making Psychotherapy Work* (Frankel, 2007), I call this development the discovery of a patient by the therapist and a therapist by the patient different from who they believe the other to be. At these points, in addition to the requirement that the therapist and patient be able to at least hear each other's perspective, there may well be a need to alter the treatment procedure as well as change the assessment measures followed, abrogating strict research protocol. For example, over time, the patient may begin to look anxious rather than depressed or show signs of hypomania not apparent earlier. Clearly, the original parameters that were followed for a clean, research-friendly treatment process may then have to go out the window, and flexibility becomes the order of the day. At these junctures, the therapist may want to call in the psychologist-assessor for extra meetings.

When I make these statements about my pessimism about adhering to a strict research design in office-based therapies like those we conduct, I am simply being realistic. Clinical work is never lacking in complexity, is rife with complications that mandate revisions in procedure, and rarely or never follows a predictable course (Westen et al., 2004).

The lack of consistency in patients' therapy requirements has its analogy in both pharmacology and general medicine. When the response to an antidepressant medication is ambiguous, we are also faced with uncertainty. We usually can't simply increase the dose of the antidepressant, add another medicine, or change the antidepressant type and be sure of getting an enduring, definitive result, but neither did increasing my Parkinson's patient Nathan's Sinemet the last time his internist saw him. It turns out that the cells of the brain stem that produce acetylcholine, the chemical neurotransmitter that is deficient in Parkinson's, were probably burning out. So the old fix didn't help. Also, Nathan was becoming discouraged and may have been missing doses of his medication either deliberately or by forgetting to take them. Again, compare medical to psychosocial treatments. Although we can often be more sure through laboratory tests of what we need to do pharmacologically in both medicine and psychiatry, in both disciplines there is always the personal and interpersonal slippage of subjectivity and the changes in clinical requirements that this factor introduces.

Doreen Continued

In contrast with her initial reluctance to become involved in treatment, Doreen agreed to 75-minute sessions twice a week and from the start came to them religiously. I also encouraged her to attend meetings of a support group for people with substance abuse problems. Here is where we encountered another therapeutic disjunction (Frankel, 2000). As dutiful as she became about attending sessions and in spite of her earnest statements about discontinuing the use of drugs, it soon became clear that Doreen would resist my view that her commitment to Bobbie seemed impulsive and was possibly misguided. She also found convoluted reasons not to attend the support group.

When Bobbie partied with her friends, Doreen would feel excluded and invariably would use drugs for a night or two along with them. One associated problem was the difficulty Doreen had being forthcoming with me about these episodes since she felt so embarrassed following them. Her promise to tell me the next time it happened was essentially hollow. Also, Doreen remained rigidly committed to the notion that Bobbie could be a life partner, unwilling to confront her on her reprehensible behavior and terrified of alienating her. Both the intermittent use of drugs and Doreen's insistence on continuing with Bobbie went on for months. These behaviors perpetuated my own dilemma of how to get beneath the surface and stop Doreen from dodging the urgency of my message that she needed to think more clearly about her reasons for continuing with Bobbie and deal with her inability to give up mind-altering chemicals.

The problem here, as I see it, is with the psychological complexity of Doreen's diagnosis. Her anxiety and depression, part of which were probably drug related, were evident. Also, Doreen was impressively self-focused, insisting that I attend to the smallest detail of her story. If I interrupted her or even got up to get writing supplies while she was talking, she became irritated. Then there was Doreen's difficulty facing the reality of Bobbie's opportunism, which had the feeling of a defect in judgment, likely resulting from her parents' egocentricity as she was growing up. There was probably a traumatic aspect as well, first brought on by weeklong abandonments by Doreen's mother during her childhood, continuing into adulthood through her disappointments in promising relationships, and, more recently, repeated in the battering she experienced through Bobbie's manipulations.

Doreen and I registered these new ideas about the etiology and complex nature of her diagnosis. Bobbie had departed abruptly months earlier, owing Doreen a considerable sum of money. Doreen allowed me to use these experiences to demonstrate how her self-absorption was making her less attractive to potential partners, thereby increasing the chance

> that she would have yet another disappointing relationship. On retesting 9 months later, it was impressive to see how significantly Doreen's neediness and anxiety had abated. Also, by this time, given what she was telling me, her effort to maintain her abstinence was intact. It is worth noting that Doreen was never able to accept referral to the support group, another imperfection in the ideal execution of our treatment.
>
> Then, without warning, Doreen's difficulties took a potentially worrisome turn. Doreen had become ambivalent about her antique business and silently reduced her level of new income-generating projects. She also made the decision to focus on her financial investments rather than the antique business since her investments had appreciated in value during an upsurge in the business cycle. As is often the case in speculative investing, however, Doreen missed the boat. Rather than continuing inexorably, the financial boom fizzled, and so did Doreen's net worth. She still had considerable assets, but she needed now to take care financially.
>
> Doreen eagerly embraced referral to a business coach I knew and whose competence and honesty I trusted. She soon realized that the neglect of her business was associated mainly with her fanatical involvement with Bobbie, the fantasy that she and Bobbie could skip blithely off into the sunset without continued attention to the details of the rest of her life. She resolved to be more cautious and to again take charge of her financial activities. Admittedly, during this period, I felt apprehensive, as Doreen worried she might not be able to afford to continue treatment. Fortunately, this concern was mitigated as she again recognized how important the therapy had been for understanding and resolving her anxiety and addiction as well as for unraveling why she was so prone to make unhealthy romantic commitments.

See appendix A at the end of this chapter for more details about the treatment phase.

Phase 4: Decision to Terminate Treatment, Posttreatment Follow-Up

The decision to terminate treatment is formulated between therapist and patient and then substantiated and guided by a full repetition of the initial testing battery. The estimated length of the termination period is a clinical decision. The traditional guideline that the duration of the termination should be roughly proportional to the duration of treatment is useful but not sacrosanct.

The first step in ending a therapy is for the therapist and patient to discuss the clinical advisability of stopping and how quickly it should happen. However, at this point, often patients are impatient to stop, insisting that since things are better, continuing to meet will only drag them down. At this point, the therapist risks becoming an adversary if he or she doesn't comply with the patient's time frame. Forcing the issue is usually counterproductive after the therapist clarifies the clinical reasons for suggesting a particular time period for ending. Further, it is not unusual for patients to balk at the idea of repeating a full battery of tests at this point. After all, they are expensive, and the retesting may feel like an unwelcomed prolongation of the therapy at just the time the patient wants it to finish.

It is also worth noting that in some treatments—and especially in work with adolescents and young adults—the desire for separation from the therapist may be developmentally appropriate. After all, emancipation from the family may be in order at that point, and leaving therapy may be required as well. The same can be said for adults who have been pathologically dependent on others and need to try their own wings.

So what happens to our research objective of collecting useful outcome data when there are so many deviations from the Center's protocol as the work progresses? Obviously, in many or even most cases, the independent variables defining that particular treatment, such as frequency of visits, therapist technique, or the involvement of others such as family members, are impossible to maintain as clinical requirements change.

The proof of whether a therapy is successful must then be in the clinical pudding, not from the clean completion of a research protocol. If the therapy works, not only will the psychometric testing show it, but patient and therapist, when not defensive, are almost certain to have their own clinical evidence to support the test findings as well. There will be a shared sense of having done a good job together. Therapy goals will appear realized or seem more approachable. Further, the results should endure, and the outcome is likely to be evident in follow-up testing. After all, that is how Dori (see chapter 1) felt as a result of her therapy with Dr. Crane but not as a result of her work with either Thea, her first psychotherapist, or, Wanda, the psychiatrist she saw just after beginning graduate school. According to Dori, treatment with Thea helped her regain balance after a disorienting postcollege experience. Also, at the end of her work with Thea, Dori felt like remaining in contact with her. For a while, she defended the experience with Thea, insisting that she was smart, not corrupted by her authority or the money she was earning from Dori's parents. Fortunately, by increments, this idealization fell away, and Dori became more realistic about Thea's limitations. Nonetheless, she acknowledges that the therapy with Thea did help. In contrast with Dr. Crane and even Thea, after Wanda refused to continue their work, Dori was simply glad to get away, left to question her own validity and stagger as she licked her wounds.

Doreen

Doreen has requested that we cut sessions down to once a week as soon as our current major retesting confirms that the change is clinically judicious. She has progressed impressively in most of the areas we established as foci for our work. She still does not have a committed romantic relationship but is much more comfortable with this state of affairs. Anxiety continues to plague her (although it is milder and less constant), she has stopped using illicit drugs, and while she has cut back, she has not yet embarked on a dedicated plan to discontinue the medication she uses for sleep and anxiety.

In order to illustrate the variety of courses a termination can take, two other case examples follow.

Deborah

My work with Deborah, a married 45-year-old mother of one grown son and a psychotherapist herself, provides an illustration of a typical termination from a less intensive yet long-term, psychodynamically oriented psychotherapy.

Deborah and I had been almost continually productive in our therapy of 3 years, she a veteran of two previous, reportedly successful therapies. Abandoned to her grandmother by remarkably insensitive parents when she was 2 years old, she was an impressive study in resilience.

Prior to our work, she was always fighting. She was careful not to let anyone, especially men, get the upper hand in relationships. She knew how insensitive people could be and was clear that no one would ever do that to her again.

That's about where we started. For her, the barrier she used to keep people at a manageable distance was actually easier for me to breach than Deborah believed it would be. She had convinced herself that her personal world was relatively impenetrable. However, the moment she walked into my office, Deborah expressed concern that I would see something to criticize about her, a worry that, in spite of her hard demeanor, left her open and approachably vulnerable. In fact, because of her past therapies, she sought and could take more scrutiny than many new patients. She did not balk when in response to her self-conscious anxiety I began talking about her false self, her wish to impress, and how these postures seemed to obscure the moment-by-moment authenticity of our encounter.

This kind of microscopic examination became the hallmark of our work. Deborah's intention was to be open and rigorous about the exploratory aspect of our once-a-week therapy. Her ability to do that was only muted by her insistence that I not carelessly reopen the painful experiences of neglect and abandonments of her childhood. Dreams, which she assiduously wrote down and examined, were always about this topic, portraying her as defective, even repulsive, causing people to avoid her.

So, after reworking her early traumas and affirming her many personal and professional successes as well as helping her consolidate her marriage, she again, after 3 years of treatment, felt ready to be on her own.

In contrast to many terminations, this one followed a traditional sequence. At first, there was the return of her original anxieties about being unacceptable to me. Typically, terminations of this sort begin with presenting symptoms returning. Deborah worried that I, like her father, would want to hang on to her for my own emotional and even financial needs. Of course, she also anticipated missing me as she did her parents when as a young child they left her with her grandparents for 6 months at a time. Finally, she wondered whether she could do as good a job on her own as we had done. And so with these considerations in mind and at her election to terminate, we took a full three and a half months to finish things off.

Deborah's initial anxiety about managing on her own yielded in about a month. Then began a period of testing me to see whether I meant it when I said I would still be here for her if she needed me again. For several weeks, she found herself arguing with her husband and for the first time in years worrying that the marriage might fail. She also had troubling dreams of being lost and not being able to find either me or her husband. Toward the end of our work, her personal barrier, her toughness, was again there, but much attenuated as compared to when we started our work. She and I talked exhaustively about the recurrence of this block to intimacy, she having recognized that its influence on her relationships was worth watching. Incidentally, I recommended that she refrain from recontacting me for about 3 months after we stopped. Both of us agreed that she should try her own wings first.

Follow-up has occurred for 2 years, and Deborah' gains have held steadily both clinically and according to the testing we continued to use. She had requested that the follow-up testing initially be limited to the PAI and TAT, citing her desire to not get "reentangled" by the therapy so soon after termination. The testing confirmed improvement in Deborah's "capacity for and interest in self-reflection, interpersonal relationships, and a significant reduction in self criticism." She has not initiated therapeutic contact on her own.

Dori

Contrasting with this example is Dori's 5-year experience in her public health graduate program and its relationship to the end of her treatment with Dr. Crane. After being in graduate school for 3 years, Dori's parents told her that they could no longer afford to pay for her psychotherapy and would be able to support only intermittent meetings with a psychopharmacologist who was on Dori's insurance plan.

Throughout the first few years of her program, Dori's professors tended to be aloof and academically severe, a style that clashed with Dori's. It was only after she finished her basic training and began an internship where her humility and decency were valued that she truly began to thrive. In evaluating the success of this experience, she refers especially to the personal relationships she established with her new supervisors. For the first time in years, Dori found herself feeling excited and happy. She says she now works 60 "satisfying" hours a week. She is clear that this dramatic shift is not the work of either psychotherapy or psychotropic medication.

Nonetheless, Dori feels deeply grateful to Dr. Crane for comprehending who she really is and not letting her own needs for control and authority get in the way of Dori's growth. She believes it was Dr. Crane's gracious way of letting go, but making clear to Dori that she will be there whenever Dori needs her mattered most. She adds that Dr. Crane says an occasional call from her just to say hello will be "most welcome."

Looking Back

In reconsidering the assessment and monitoring measures we have recommended, we believe that the need for flexibility—the willingness to alter one's treatment plan, tactics, and style in accordance with the therapist's and patient's clinical judgment and feedback from testing—is mandatory in clinical work. Research interests, although admirable, often need to be shelved in deference to clinical judgment. I realize that to at least some of the more research minded among us, the notion of modifying a therapy procedure according to clinical judgment may seem like a corruption of standards. But, in fact, as clinicians we have no alternative. Our goal is to do our part to help untangle people themselves from their inevitably complicated personal and psychological dilemmas. Further, we are convinced that our method needs to be practical so that it can and will be used by therapists in their offices with the entire range of psychotherapy patients they treat.

Onward

Our next task is to reframe the Center's procedures so that they can be used for children and adolescents. Work within this age range should always be considered developmentally specific. Developmental considerations add not only to the complexity of assessing and treating children and adolescents but also to its fascination. In my experience, a heightened sense of promise is typical in work with these age-groups. One can expect results with children and adolescents to come faster and be more clearly life changing than with adults. Finally, the technical challenge of this work involves ongoing collaboration with parents and often teachers as well as other supporting figures; such collaboration is necessary since children and even adolescents are still usually quite dependent on parents for financial and emotional support.

Appendix A

I. Information to Be Gathered During the Clinical Evaluation and Projected Time Allocations:

a. Screening call

Information to be recorded:

Referral source

Basic data including:

name, address, telephone numbers (mother's and father's if the patient is a child), birth date, marital status, including number of marriages, occupation or in school, children, siblings, dates and reasons for the most recent psychiatric interventions, medications, and ongoing medical treatments.

Reasons for referral:

Who is informant(s)? Is patient's reason for coming different from parents', from referring agency?

Fee (discussed? with whom?)

(time for the screening call: 30 minutes)

II. Materials given or sent to patient or parents either preceding or following the initial meeting:

Fee agreement

Basic information sheet

Personal data and history organizers (child or adult, long or short version?): Added may be standard history and/or self-report inventories addressing specific problems such as attention deficit disorder or depression.

Permissions to speak to relevant individuals or agencies and requests for records: sent and when?

III. The initial meeting:
(75 to 90 minutes)

This may simply be a screening meeting for the parents and the patient. Referral to other professionals for treatment is possible at this point. The purpose of this meeting is for the patient (and the parents in the case of a child or adolescent) to form an initial impression of the therapist and to begin to discuss treatment options. Included is time for answering the parents' and patient's questions about the evaluation, the treatment process, and the therapist's credentials, professional orientation, and personal background.

At this meeting, if possible, the therapist and patient begin to use the Target Complaint and Goal Attainment questionnaires and any other appropriate self-report inventories to develop an ongoing, formal record of the patient's difficulties. Note: If the work-up is of a child or an adolescent, the child (and in most cases the adolescent) is usually excluded from this meeting.

To the extent that the patient is not able or willing to complete personal history forms, the therapist will need to gather this information by interview.

IV. Beyond the initial meeting:

a. Sessions 2 to 5: Clinical data gathering and contacting collateral sources of information continues; therapist and patient begin to develop a working relationship. At the end of this phase, there is a wrap-up session. Tentative recommendations and treatment options are processed by patient and therapist. The treatment plan, after it is developed, is revised periodically in collaboration with the patient. The therapist also reviews pertinent records, including past psychological testing, medical records, and school records.

b. There may be meetings with the patient's spouse or other significant people in the patient's life, as needed and appropriate. If the patient is a child or adolescent home and school visit(s) may be arranged.

(time: two to four 75- to 90-minute sessions, plus time speaking to informants and outside consultants, school or home visits when assessing and treating adolescents and children, and extra meetings as required.)

i. Child and adolescent evaluations are explained in chapter 6. These specialized workups typically require one or two meetings with parents (as well as one extra if needed for orientation) and two to four meetings with child plus possible home and/or school visit.

c. The therapist begins to contact collateral sources of information either by phone or in person. Included are others who have had close contact with or evaluated the patient, including tutors, nannies, teachers, medical doctors, or family members. (time: undetermined, usually 1 to 2 hours)

V. The Second, Testing Phase of the Initial Evaluation:

Information to be gathered during the testing phase and projected time required at each step:

a. The psychologist-assessor enters the treatment field when clinically indicated, usually 4 to 12 weeks into the evaluation or initial treatment. This aspect of the evaluation usually takes 1 to 2 months. Note: The psychologist-assessor's charges are separate from the therapist's.

The evaluation by the psychologist-assessor is conducted collaboratively with the therapist and patient. Both therapist and patient submit questions they would like the psychologist-assessor to address in writing and, when they desire, comments about treatment. The testing involves the assessment batteries described in Appendix B.

Ideally, a feedback meeting takes place 6 to 12 weeks from the inception of the evaluation and includes the psychologist-assessor, patient, and therapist.

The steps in this part of the assessment are as follows:

i. Phone discussion between therapist and the psychologist-assessor. The psychologist-assessor and therapist should at least discuss the therapist's goals for the consultation.

ii. Initial meeting(s) between the psychologist-assessor, patient, and possibly the therapist. (time for therapist's participation: 50 to 90 minutes)

iii. Therapist and patient submit questions and, when desired, comments in writing to the psychologist-assessor. These inquiries need to be frank and include questions to be addressed in testing as well as concerns about the treatment.

iv. The initial meetings between the psychologist-assessor and patient allow for a clinical evaluation by the psychologist-assessor. He or she also needs to decide which testing instruments to use and how to schedule these.

v. Neuropsychological or Psychological Testing.
vi. Testing is followed by one or more feedback sessions. The feedback begins a collaborative planning process involving therapist and patient, and at times include the psychologist-assessor.
vii. As possible, retesting is done at 6-month intervals using the testing schedule described previously. A full retesting is repeated approximately every 18 months. These contacts should include resubmission of questions to the psychologist assessor by both the patient and the therapist, and except at the time of a major testing, at least a follow-up phone call between the psychologist-assessor and therapist. Whether there should be a formal feedback meeting involving the therapist, patient, and psychologist-assessor is decided on a case-by-case basis. The psychologist-assessor's impressions and findings should be verbal and in writing.

VI. All Phases: Instruments Used for The Initial Assessment and Treatment Monitoring
a. Frequently: The therapist and patient complete the Target Complaint and Goal Attainment Questionnaires every two to four weeks. The therapist takes notes during each session.
b. For adults, the psychologist-assessor administers an abbreviated or full Wechsler Scale of Intelligence (WISC for children, WAIS for adults), PAI, SCL-90, Neuropsychological Impairment Scale (NIS), and Rorschach. Approximately every 6 months thereafter, the psychologist-assessor readministers a PAI, SCL-90, NIS, and any other self-report inventories specific to the patient's problems, such as the Beck or Hamilton anxiety or depression scales, or the Conners' or Gordon Systems tests of attention. Once every 18 months and a few months before the planned end of treatment, he or she repeats the original testing battery. Note that the full WISC or WASI take vastly more time than the abbreviated versions. The full versions also provide a good deal more information beyond estimating intelligence.

The original psychologist-assessor remains involved throughout the treatment if possible. Each meeting with the psychologist-assessor is conducted collaboratively with some form of communication between him- or herself and the patient and therapist, separately or together. The timing of this ongoing testing and consultation is flexible and based partially on whether its inclusion in treatment at that point is likely to impede or facilitate the treatment process. There is at least one feedback session after each major testing and a phone call between psychologist-assessor, patient, and therapist separately when less extensive testing is done. A report is written by the psychologist-assessor and included in the patient's record after major testing and, if possible, after 6-month reassessments. Additional collaborative meetings with the psychologist-assessor and the patient and therapist, either alone or together, should be scheduled as needed.

c. Other consultants in areas such as education or vocational counseling are engaged as needed. Reports are requested.
d. A medical examination, including appropriate diagnostic tests, is done at the beginning of treatment and approximately yearly thereafter. Note that as part of the initial screen, basic medical information is requested from the patient.

Appendix B: Summary of Tests Used in a Model Center Evaluation of an Adult

Initially and then every 6 months: the PAI, the SCL-90, the NIS, and possibly the NEO Personality Inventory are administered. Initially, again every 18 months or so, and then several months before the end of treatment: the WAIS or WASI (full or abbreviated versions) depending on whether the patient is a child, the Rorschach Test.

This list is somewhat different for children and adolescents and may be modified by adding tests targeting particular problem areas. For example, attention deficit disorder can be highlighted by inventories such as the Gordon System or the Conners' Continuous Performance Test, while executive function problems require the use of assessments evaluating the patient's capacity to plan and organize such as the Wisconsin Card Sort Test, the Tower of London, and Delis-Kaplan tests of executive function. Note also that the patient's cognitive functioning can be approximated by a brief screening instrument such as the Wechsler Abbreviated Scale of Intelligence. The entire WAIS for adults or the Wechsler Intelligence Scale for Children (WISC) can be added. A full WISC or WAIS is more informative but adds extra time and cost to the evaluation.

Other tests assessing interpersonal interest and capacity can be added as needed. This group includes the Thematic Apperception Test (TAT), the Roberts Apperception Test for children and adolescents, the Scale of Interpersonal Problems, and the Adult Attachment Projective.

CHAPTER SIX

Our Methods and Procedures: Children and Adolescents

This chapter is a sequel to chapter 5 describing the Center for Collaborative Psychology and Psychiatry's assessment and monitoring procedures for adults. It adds two new categories: children, who I will define as being from preschool age through early puberty, approximately between 10 and 13 years of age, and adolescents, ranging in age from the early teens through the mid-20s and even early 30s.

Developmental considerations create unique requirements and opportunities. Child and adolescent work is almost always more multifaceted than that with adults. In addition to maturational and developmental considerations, impacting the treatment also are the child's or adolescent's cultural milieu, family, and school. While complex in their requirements, children and adolescents offer endless interesting clinical possibilities. Because children are so dependent on their parents or caretakers, the authority of parents, teachers, and therapists is usually more decisive in work with them than for adults. Perhaps, surprisingly, the same is often true for adolescents, who remain more dependent on their parents than they generally like to acknowledge. Intelligently planning a child- or adolescent-oriented intervention requires collaboration with and guidance from parents, engaging them as critical supports to the treatment.

My point so far has been to distinguish the technical challenge of assessment and treatment of children and adolescents from that for work with adults. While both age-groups require a committed relationship with a therapist for the therapy to succeed, ground rules for understanding and treating the younger patient are often vastly different than those for adults (Fonagy, Target, Cottrell, Phillips, & Kurtz, 2002). The capacities, interests, and support systems of children and adolescents are unique to their personal and developmental status. Distress and psychopathology is expressed differently by children than it is by adults, more often behaviorally. The ability of children and even of adolescents to plan and conceptualize is more limited than it is for adults despite the fuller emergence of these capabilities during adolescence.

Differentiating Children and Adults

Psychopathology

Children and adolescents are not physiologically or psychologically miniature adults (Sroufe, Egeland, Carlson, & Collins, 2005). Nor is their psychopathology a reduced version of that which afflicts adults (Fonagy et al., 2002). In addition to their continued dependence on adult support, children and adolescents are developmentally unfinished, grappling with issues different from those occupying adults. In turn, entities arising during childhood or becoming problematic during adolescence generally require remedial measures different than those used for adults.

Begin with entities that are on the borderline between the psychological and the physiological and their fate. How do you know whether attention deficit disorder or a conduct disorder will persist into adulthood and what form it will take? Will a conduct disorder turn into sociopathy and eventuate in endless unstable relationships or the inability to hold a job? Are episodes of disorganization or even blatant lapses into fantasy necessarily the harbinger of adult schizophrenia or even adult borderline personality disorder?

Then there are developmental disorders such as Asperger's syndrome. These may be amenable to socialization therapy but regardless of psychological sequelae are not psychologically based, and therefore their essential remediation is not responsive to conventional psychotherapy. Left out are the ever-present constitutionally based learning disabilities, some of which can be crippling and create crises of confidence for the child that are never overcome.

The multiplicity of developmental anomalies that are so disabling in childhood are paralleled in variety and ubiquity only by subtle neurological disorders that determine whether a child or adolescent will be able to meet developmental challenges. Witness, for example, fetal alcohol syndrome, which can be brought about by a mother consuming even small amounts of alcohol during the first trimester of pregnancy. Nonverbal learning disability, by now well accepted as a neuropsychological condition, is another hard-to-diagnose entity frequently correlated with social problems characterized by an inability to read social cues.

Developmental disorders can have a biological etiology, an environmental etiology, or both. Environmentally caused "developmental" disorders of early childhood include problems with attachment, which, unlike the autistic-spectrum entities like Asperger's, are often based on trauma or deprivation. Finally, latent adult major depressive disorder or bipolar disorder often is mistaken in childhood or even adolescence to be a temperamental idiosyncrasy and the actual diagnosis missed until much later.

Treatment

Treatment methods for disorders of childhood and adolescence also differ from those for adults. The unique technical requirements for planning and implementing child or adolescent treatment identify an area of therapeutic expertise all its own. Certainly, behavioral measures and cognitive restructuring techniques are often useful with both age-groups. But reparenting, environmental engineering that usually relies on work with parents, educational measures, and socialization treatments are infrequently selected as treatment modalities in adult work. Insight-oriented psychotherapy with children differs from its counterpart with adults. Metaphor and play, rather than words, are the medium of children's thinking and communication. Competent use of these vehicles therapeutically requires specialized training and experience.

Unique measures are required in work with children and even adolescents whose development has been arrested because of the psychological impact of parental neglect or incompetence (Kagan, 1997; Sroufe et al., 2005). Delayed socialization or impaired capacity for empathy are common manifestations of these disorders. Here the relationship with the therapist itself may correct for missed or distorted parenting. While a version of this reparenting experience often takes place implicitly in psychotherapy with adults, the parental impact of a psychotherapist is likely to be more explicit and instrumental in work with a child or adolescent who him- or herself is in the throes of development. Often, more important, the reparenting work may be done by the parents themselves. Here the therapist provides guidance or, perhaps more aptly, coaching for the parents, putting them back on track with their child or adolescent. This approach prepares the therapist to progressively exit the family arena, leaving family business, appropriately, to the more competent and empowered set of parents.

Children: How Malleable?

My statements reflect the conviction that, compared to adults, children through childhood and adolescence tend to be especially capable of spontaneously revising and even reversing emotional problems and developmental arrests. Regarding change through talk or play therapy, especially up to about age 7, children have limited capacity for self-reflection. They also are developmentally egocentric (Flavell, 1963), putting a cap on their capacity for empathy and ability to understand the needs and motivations of others. Psychotherapy with this age-group needs to be configured according to these kinds of developmentally specific emotional tolerances and cognitive limitations.

Contrasting with situations where the interpersonal impact of the relationship is central to its therapeutic power are those where the child's or adolescent's problems are constitutionally based. Included are pervasive developmental disorders, specific and nonverbal learning disabilities, and the spectrum of attentional disorders. Within this diagnostic range, educational and pediatric consultations are likely to be especially valuable in devising a useful treatment.

General Considerations

There is hardly a child or adolescent therapy in which the therapist is not legitimately accountable to parents. In fact, when treating a child or even an adolescent, work with parents is sometimes all that is required to achieve the desired result. The therapist meets with the child or adolescent in these cases mainly for diagnostic purposes. In keeping with this thinking, my model for psychotherapy with adolescents allows for significant involvement between therapist and parents. My viewpoint differs sharply with the tradition of minimizing parent contact in adolescent treatment or keeping them out of it altogether. Added to parents, child assessment and adolescent treatment frequently requires collateral work with teachers, tutors, nannies, and pediatricians.

A related consideration is confidentiality, especially in work with adolescents. While there is hardly a child or an adolescent who will not overtly object to the therapist telling details of therapy conversations to parents, nonetheless not sharing may reflect poor judgment, impeding therapeutic progress as the parents grow distant from the therapy. In these cases, the clinical dilemma may actually become whether the therapist should also share with the child or adolescent the details of his or her subsequent contact with the parents. Deciding not to confide in parents, especially when the child's or adolescent's behavior is worrisome, almost always creates an ethical and even legal quandary for the therapist. Yet telling everything may be counterproductive, eroding the child's or adolescent's trust in the therapist.

What should I have done, for example, when I learned that Chad, an adolescent-like 23-year-old fifth-year college dilettante, was not just using Ecstasy every weekend but had organized a ring of drug dealers at his school? Chad's parents were fine people, fervently concerned about their son's welfare. However, their preoccupation with their careers and with their developmentally disabled older son took up most of their time. Chad was sidelined from the time he could talk. Their solution to their time dilemma was to send Chad to boarding school and to give him everything he wanted materially. Then when he was 12, they divorced and threw Chad's life into even more serious disarray. Chad had no choice. He had to fend for himself and of necessity became opportunistic. For example, one lesson Chad learned well was how to hit his mother up for money and privileges while doing the same with his father. He also became a master liar, able to create any believable story that would get him what he wanted.

So you can probably live with my judiciously snitching on Chad to the parents. After all, he was frittering away his young life, and both the parents were impeccably trustworthy. But what about my relationship with Chad? Should I have told him everything about my conversations with, including my advice to, his parents? Chad absolutely trusted me. He knew he lived a life of deception and believed he was in trouble. He actually craved the involvement and direction his parents had failed to provide earlier. Yet like most adolescents, he vociferously objected to their regulating his life.

There are, of course, many other considerations in framing a successful treatment strategy with a child or an adolescent. A few precautionary measures include the following.

In child treatment and in some adolescent cases, a behavioral regime prescribing the most developmentally appropriate remedial measures for the parents, teachers, and therapist to follow is almost always formulated. Medications are prescribed as required.

Also to be considered are the child's—and particularly the adolescent's—need to be with peers. As much as possible, therapy appointments should be timed so that they do not interfere with a child's social development or an adolescent's social calendar. This consideration, peer relationships, mandates that therapy appointments not be so frequent that they compete with the child's or adolescent's social life. In short, too much therapy as well as poorly timed appointments can as much impede as facilitate a child's movement toward health.

At the Center, we strive to take full responsibility for each case. In phase 1, using assessment instruments and clinical interviews, we make a comprehensive evaluation. Phase 2, which is actually part of the initial assessment, involves testing and the formulation of a treatment plan. Phase 3 consists of treatment of whatever sort and frequency is indicated. Referral to other professionals, including educational experts, is always a possibility. If we do the treatment, we work with the patient and psychologist-assessor to collaboratively monitor progress and revise procedures as needed. We are always ready for surprises and willing to change course in accordance with new information and the patient's revised needs. Phase 4 is marked by the decision to terminate treatment, and its timing is confirmed by a repeat of the initial testing battery. Phase 5, following termination, consists of interviews and assessments to confirm that treatment gains have held and to provide whatever continuing input the patient desires.

Phase 1: The Initial Clinical Assessment of a Child

The initial clinical assessment is conducted by the therapist-evaluator and usually requires one or more history-taking sessions with the parents, including a review of the child's clinical and school records. One or two meetings with parents and two to four clinical meetings with the child follow. Parents may be present in these meetings if needed to facilitate the evaluation. It is often judicious to call parents following one or more of these meetings to assure them that the evaluation is on track or to ask for more information. Home and school visits by the therapist and later in the evaluation, possibly by the psychologist who does the testing, may be helpful. Often a phone call to the child's pediatrician and almost always to teachers is indicated.

Initial Tasks

An initial telephone conversation gives the parents an opportunity to ask the therapist basic questions, discuss how fees are charged, and be introduced to the Center's procedures. The parents or parent are also referred to our website for biographical information about us and the way we practice. Initial appointments are made. The child or adolescent is usually excluded from the first visit or two.

If the patient is a child, data sheets containing basic information, a record of contact with other professionals, and personal and family history are completed, almost always by parents alone. Parents and teachers, and when possible, the child complete history and symptom checklists. Self-report history and symptom questionnaires as well as behavioral inventories are distributed to teachers and filled out by the parents and child if appropriate. When a therapist version is available, the therapist completes complementary forms.

Outcome of Initial Clinical Assessment

The therapist develops an initial case formulation with a tentative diagnostic impression involving personality, psychosocial, and biological, including medical and generic, factors; works it over with the parents; and begins to engage the child. In child and occasionally in adolescent cases, as mentioned previously, work with parents and teachers may be all that is required to begin to move the patient along. Taking this stance assumes that the therapist can verify his or her impressions of the issues that need to be dealt with through meetings with the child or adolescent and through the Center's assessment procedures discussed earlier. As part of this work-up, the family's ability and willingness to afford the evaluation and ongoing treatment, as well as the child's support systems, must be factored in. Single and divorced parents may require special financial and scheduling measures, all of which should be in place by the end of this initial phase of the assessment. The evaluator identifies data still to be collected to arrive at a definitive determination of goals and procedures. Included should be a list of informants to be contacted and additional categories of information required, as well as assessments still to be done and by whom they will be carried out. Consultants, especially in the field of education or childhood developmental disorders, may need to be called in.

At the end of this period, parents should be fully informed of the Center's procedures, especially the testing protocol we use to confirm diagnosis and monitor progress. A tentative agreement to begin treatment should be made. These guidelines are shared with the child and especially the adolescent to the extent that they apply to and can be comprehended by him or her. However, it is the parents who are the ultimate support for the treatment, and at this point in the initial clinical assessment, it is their commitment that is most critical. There is literally no child or, for that matter, adolescent treatment that can survive for long without parental backing. One or both parents can subtly undermine a treatment by even nonverbally communicating their disapproval to their child. The erosive effect of this communication eventually becomes manifest in the child or parent losing interest in the treatment or actively sabotaging it.

It needs to be clear to parents that even at this point, critical historical, psychological, and sociological data may still be missing and will have to be gleaned by the therapist over time. I am referring here to information that family members may consider proprietary, such as acknowledging that there is marital discord or information that parents or even the therapist may at first think is unimportant, such as about the grief experienced after a series of miscarriages just before the patient's birth. Final determination of the length and frequency of visits is delayed until the first testing battery is completed. Plans for testing may be postponed for an undetermined period until the parents understand its purpose and accept its value. While the child's or adolescent's permission may not be required for testing to proceed, his or her cooperation is usually required for the testing to be valid. At the very least, he or she will need to understand the purpose of the testing and how it will be administered. Ideally, he or she should feel reasonably assured of its potential benefit to him or her.

Note that parents often want the therapist to make predictions about the duration of treatment. While this request is usually justified, it is important to convey to parents that this prediction will become reliable only as the treatment progresses and as the capacities and tolerances of the child and parents are made clear. Also, treatment length will in part depend on the resources and time the parents are willing to allocate to the treatment and the collateral work supporting it. Nonetheless, the request that the therapist estimate the length and time of a treatment must be acknowledged and addressed to the best of the therapist's and psychologist-evaluator's ability.

A requirement of this phase of the assessment is the formulation of goals and development of a formal plan of action that may include the patient's entire support system, including parents and teachers. If possible, this plan should be developed and implemented with the cooperation of the patient. Alternatively, the decision for referral to another psychotherapist or allied professional may be made. After all, the Center—its personnel and resources—may not fit or be able to accommodate everyone's needs.

In my experience, psychotherapy with children and adolescents often derives much of its power from the therapist's indirect influence implemented through parents, teachers, and other people important to the patient. A therapist may find him- or herself believing that the technical power of his or her intervention is responsible for the lion's share of the child's improvement. Instead, a shift in the parents' attitude toward more involvement with the child or support from others, such as a respected teacher or a coach, may be the most influential factor. In fact, creating a more competent set of parents is often key to a child's progress. Continued growth may be facilitated by environmental supplementation put in place by the parents and therapist during treatment. For example, Damien, who will be discussed later, became a new person soon after his parents enrolled him in tae kwon do martial arts training. His vision problems had made it impossible for him to successfully participate in ball sports.

Regarding the power of the therapy itself, clinically one often observes the child forming a powerful bond with the therapist and seizing on it to move forward. A careful analysis of the factors responsible for this change often reveals that the relationship with the therapist was decisive and that insight had little to do with it. Instead, the therapist, like a good parent, has guided or inspired, providing the technical and emotional support the child needed to progress.

Phase 2: Testing, Feedback, and Reformulation of the Plan

This phase is broached when the parents (and, if possible, the patient) and the therapist are able to formulate accurate testing questions. This part of the assessment procedure is the same as with adults. By this point, the parents and patient have usually formed their initial impressions of the therapist and therapy. When pertinent, comments about their impressions are submitted in writing along with the testing questions. Testing is initiated.

The psychologist-assessor needs to tentatively determine which test parameters and protocols to follow. Revisions may be required, however, as treatment progresses, mandating that the procedures and tests used for ongoing diagnosis and monitoring change.

Phase 3: Treatment Proper

Psychotherapy is paced and structured through clinical and formal determinations of treatment progress. When progress slows or stops, the psychologist-assessor often is called back. Always at issue are the child's or adolescent's psychological and developmental needs as well as the therapist's accuracy. These considerations may at times dictate radical revisions in the measures that the treatment team decides are in the patient's best interest. For example, a period of conjoint treatment with the parents or even a sibling, family therapy, or a decrease or increase in the frequency of sessions may be implemented. The therapist may need to seek outside consultation to clarify where he or she is failing or succeeding with the patient.

Collaboration with school, tutors, and nannies is almost always required in treatment of children. Regular visits with parents are as well.

Phase 4: Decision to Restrict or End Treatment

In addition to clinical judgment based on the therapist's opinion and the patient's and parents' wishes, support for the decision to restrict or stop treatment should ideally come from another round of testing supported by the clinical observations of the psychologist-assessor and, if relevant, observations from teachers and others who have been involved in the treatment. Tests used here are selected as much for convenience as for comprehensiveness since the decision to terminate treatment in a child or adolescent is usually made in deference to the patient's current needs and frame of mind about continuing and less according to an established testing schedule. The questions to be answered are usually more clearly tied to the patient's life circumstances than in adult treatment and may be well enough addressed by the Behavior Assessment System for Children (BASC) or either the Personality Inventory for Children or the Personality Inventory for Youth. Nonetheless, as much as possible, a formal period of termination should be planned.

Two or 3 months before ending, the psychologist-assessor administers a full battery of psychological or neuropsychological tests. As nearly as possible, the final testing battery should replicate the one given at the beginning of treatment. However, a full battery is often not acceptable to the patient or his or her parents at this point, especially if they are looking forward to therapy ending. Frequently, retesting suggests to them that the therapist intends to prolong treatment. Also, as mentioned, extending treatment may be especially problematic for a late adolescent or young adult who is developmentally poised to take control of his or her life.

Criteria for success in treatment with children and adolescents is not necessarily the same as in work with adults. In psychotherapy with children and adolescents, the focus is not as likely to be on the full resolution of symptoms and problematic behaviors. Returning the patient to a normal developmental trajectory is often most appropriate and of at least equal importance given the child's developmental needs. From this point, development itself may provide what the patient requires to move ahead. Termination of treatment is often undertaken with the child developmentally unfinished, still in the process of changing. It is not unusual for the therapist to be convinced that a child—and especially an adolescent—needs more work while recognizing that keeping him or her in therapy will actually entrap him or her. These considerations make previous experience working with these age-groups especially relevant when undertaking a termination with a child or an adolescent.

The therapist terminating with an improved but as-yet-unfinished child or adolescent patient is in an interesting position, one not often encountered in work with adults. He or she is acutely aware that his or her power to predict is limited. There is no way to know what turns development will take. This observation in itself is a good argument for therapist humility. In fact, the truest and most productive course for the work at this point is to keep the jury out while capitalizing on gains made in therapy to date. The therapist adopts a wait-and-see attitude in cooperation with the parents, checking in periodically to see if a tune-up is called for. In this way, the developing child or adolescent, together with the parents, has the best shot at taking the most productive and creative trajectory possible.

Phase 5: Follow-Up After Termination

Ideally, the therapist him- or herself should carry out follow-up. The therapist's familiarity with the patient and parents is likely to be invaluable in understanding the limited data available from follow-up interviews and testing. When possible, formal reassessment, usually using our briefer testing protocol, should occur for at least 2 to 4 years posttreatment and be repeated every 9 to 18 months. To the degree that the parents or patient feel that posttermination adjustment and progress would be violated by testing, these reassessments may simply have to consist of discussions between the parents (and, if possible, the patient) and the therapist in person or by phone and, when available, the completion by them of self-assessment inventories. Periodic telephone calls to parents, if only to express ongoing interest, are usually appreciated, making their continued cooperation more likely. When available, contacts with the patient's teachers may also provide helpful follow-up information.

Case Example: Damien

At age 10, Damien and his family indeed were a diagnostic and treatment morass. Can you imagine being called into the vice principal's office no less than three times a week? While you are contrite each time this happens, you lose it again the next day when a girl inadvertently steps on your foot in the midst of some mild, age-appropriate teasing at recess.

Even worse were the less frequent, wilder moments, such as the one at a family gathering when Damien's 2-year-old cousin got into his action cards and messed them up. According to Damien, his mother defended his cousin, and Damien went into a rage, uncontrollably screaming that he wanted to kill his little cousin and that she could have stopped herself from messing up his cards had she wanted to. Why, he wondered with complete consternation, did she not apply the same standards of behavior to the cousin as to him? The age difference wasn't important, according to Damien. His mother, as so often in the past, was simply being unfair.

And yet, confusingly, Damien was smart and thoughtful when not emotionally overwrought. He had kind of a Harry Potter mind, never failing to produce flashes of brilliance. Oh yes, and he was always, always intent on doing the right thing. It was just that often he suddenly lost his temper in spite of his best intentions.

Admittedly, being in the fifth grade, Damien was edging up to preadolescence. Physically and emotionally, however, he was still very much a child. His room was that of a latency boy's, action and sports cards everywhere. He was not interested in sexuality and was often the butt of teasing admiration by the girls during their daily four-square games at school breaks. Because of his outbursts, he had no friends. The other children were confused by and afraid of him. He had no recourse other than to see them as unimportant and claim, defensively of course, that he didn't care even if they hated him. After all, his inability to predict and control his rages made it likely that he would never have any friends.

Damien's single most pressing wish was for his mother to reunite with his father, who lived 800 miles away in Phoenix. His mother had moved with Damien and his 2-years-younger sister to San Francisco soon after the divorce when Damien was 5. Both his mother and his father were nice people and cooperated after the divorce. In fact, the divorce was a welcome relief from their savage arguing earlier. To make matters worse, Damien's mother, who was in real estate and renovated homes, had moved twice since coming to the San Francisco Bay Area. Leaving no time for Damien to gather any social moss, the moves significantly contributed to his progressively unsatisfactory social adjustment. Also, his mother had remarried 2 years before my initial contact with Damien. Damien's stepfather was a decent soul and got on well with Damien and his father. However, he understandably was a confusing factor in Damien's life. For one thing, he was employed successfully as a lawyer, a stark contrast to Damien's father, who had worked in high-level corporate management and for the past several years had been unable to find employment.

My purpose here, however, is not to provide a full clinical case example but, instead, to illustrate a Center work-up for a child under 12. In Damien's case, the previously given outline was followed with accommodation for his unique circumstances, in this case a father living 400 miles away. Since parents are the main informants in child work-ups,

Damien's father was included from the start. Complicating matters, since Damien's father was out of work, Damien's mother paid for the psychotherapy and later the testing. Damien's father, however, agreed to pay for the discussions and meetings he had with me alone. He willingly visited me on one of his monthly trips to see Damien and his sister. While he was cooperative, my judgment (as well as Damien's later on) was that he was far too emotionally superficial to understand the depth of his son's desperation about being unable to contain his rages and to be an effective part of a therapy plan.

The need for collaboration with Damien's teachers and the battered administrative staff of his school was evident right from the beginning. Not only was their input by phone and in the form of self-assessment questionnaires necessary, but so was a several-hours visit to the school. As is often the case when teachers are faced with working with a psychotherapist, until they met me, the beleaguered school officials and teacher stereotyped me as impractical and probably of little use to them.

Also, because of the frequency of his aggressive outbursts, I needed to swing into action with Damien more quickly than I might have with an adult. I prescribed Ritalin as a trial since he clearly had an attentional disorder and some kind of emotional dyscontrol syndrome. Ritalin is a good drug for clinical experimentation since it has a rapid onset, lasts for about 4 hours, has a symptomatic effect only, and then goes away. However, Ritalin may exacerbate aggression in children, and I had to begin using it gingerly. Also, while there had been myriad psychological stressors in his life to help explain them, Damien's aggressive behavior and attentional problems almost certainly had a significant biological component.

Incidentally, Damien's mother had serious attentional problems during her own childhood and adolescence that were at least in part set off by her own mother marrying four times. Nonetheless, with plenty of remedial help, she did well beginning in mid-adolescence and graduated from an excellent small college in the Midwest. Indeed, like Damien, she was smart but impossibly scattered. As another parallel to Damien, his mother was prone to rage attacks. She was easily overwhelmed by professional and parenting responsibilities. However, her rages occurred especially when Damien misbehaved. Prior to my involvement, she was distinctly unsympathetic toward Damien, amending this attitude only as she and I worked together.

Damien's mother tended toward a view of life in which wishful thinking could make problems disappear. If you didn't want them to be there, you could simply blame someone else and imagine that if that person disappeared your life would be delightful. Prior to our work together, her inability to take responsibility for Damien's problems created an impossible barrier to progress for both Damien and his by then hand-wringing teachers.

Damien's father, whose parents also had been divorced during his childhood and whose father had been a rigid, moralistic research chemist, reported no such problems. However, his level of denial and his insufferably superficial response to Damien's behavior problem proved to be distinctly less tractable than Damien's mother's inability to grapple with Damien's problems. In fact, his father's rage episodes were actually more vicious and devastating than those of his ex-wife, even though they occurred less frequently.

Because of his behavioral dyscontrol, Damien needed neuropsychological testing more quickly than is usual with adults beginning treatment. Ironically, however, the payment imbalance between Damien's mother and father delayed this process for 5 months, with Damien's mother eventually taking on the whole thing. The point here, again, is that the ground rules for strategizing an assessment and a psychotherapy with a child are often even less amenable to a formula than those with adults. Differences between orchestrating adult and child treatment include the roles that parents play as informants, in supporting the treatment, and, in Damien's case, cooperating with therapeutic strategies, such as those requiring behavior management. As with Damien, the time frame for testing and swinging into action is often briefer for a child than for an adult and, given the child's limited ability to communicate about the nature of his or her distress, more urgent. Ancillary personnel, such as teachers, also tend to play a major role in the assessment of children.

The character of the therapy relationship with children and adolescents is also different from that with adults and in some ways more confusing. Success with Damien required that I be his friend and adviser, not just his therapist. In order to listen to and collaborate with me, he had to not only trust me but like me as well. Damien's own motivation for changing was okay, but his desire to please me, wanting me to admire him as a father might, was truly powerful. With adults, compliance of this sort is typically regarded as working against self-reflection and progress. In contrast, as a child, Damien's wish to please me was highly desirable, required for the therapy to be meaningful to him. After all, because of his age, he had not fully accepted responsibility for his emotions and actions or even considered the place of self-reflection in their management. My argument is that, with Damien at age 11, there was distinctly more justification for creating a "real," even parental, relationship as a cornerstone of the psychotherapy than there might have been if he were older. Of course, I needed to be careful not to compete with Damien's parents in embracing and encouraging this kind of involvement. Also, the potential for blurring boundaries mandated that I be judicious not to overstep the bounds of my role.

As is so typical of work with children and their families, therapy with Damien and his mother and father was challengingly multifaceted. In his case, medication has played an important therapeutic role; in other child cases, it may not.

And then suddenly, not so slowly, children like Damien experience the upsurge of hormones, and presto, you have an adolescent on your hands. We were on the verge of such a upheaval with Damien, another reason why we had to work so fast.

A Comment About Adolescence

With the exception of the tests and questionnaires used, the assessment method for adolescents is a cross between that used for adults and that used for children prior to the onset of puberty. It differs from the procedure used for adults in that primarily someone other than the patient often provides historical information. Also, the nature of the therapist's ongoing collaboration with parents and teachers is more patient and age related for adolescents than for younger children.

Who Is an Adolescent?

Setting an age range for adolescence is tricky. Adolescence is officially ushered in by the onset of puberty. However, because of media and Internet exposure, adolescent-seeming sexual themes are introduced into the life of children with and before Barbie and Ken dolls. Other powerful influences include peers and at what point they happen to enter adolescence, whether or not in sync with the patient. Prior to hormone-induced changes, however, adolescent-seeming interests actually tend to be preadolescent in quality, organized around video games, collections, and friends. It is the upsurge of hormones that drives the essential shift to adolescence proper together with the changes in peer attitudes.

Regarding psychological maturity, through the middle of high school, usually at age 16 or 17, the adolescents I encounter in northern California tend to be unclear about their reasons for making a commitment to school and usually have a very limited sense of where their lives may be leading. For many adolescents, the demarcation between early and mid-adolescence is when the adolescent can begin to drive. In many states, this age is between 15 and 16. Piaget's (1954) staging generally works well here, with planning and conceptual capacities and formal operations coming into the fore at about that point and the adolescent finally able to seriously imagine a future.

Traditionally, adolescence ended in the late teens or, in the extreme, in the early to mid-20s. Today, however, the upper limit is far less clear. The transition to an adult mentality is apparently culturally bound. As the expected life span increases, technology advances, and other changes in society occur, the move to adulthood can be increasingly deferred. Its timing is often affected by affluence (Levine, 2006), cultural background, and geographical location. For example, in England, movement into adulthood seems to occur earlier for those from a working-class background than those whose parents are university educated (statement issued by New Dynamics of Ageing Programme of the UK, a collaboration between UK's Research Councils). College for American youth is often more like a moratorium (Erikson, 1968) than a time preparing for and grappling with life. As a result of these biological and sociological shifts, it is not uncommon for people to wait until their mid-30s or even late 30s before making a commitment to a romantic partnership and profession. Until that time, they may remain dependent on parents for partial support and even move in and out of their parents' home.

Contributing also are changes in reproductive technology. As they approach their fifth decade, women who want children still need to worry about an increasing incidence of birth defects. But these can increasingly be detected in utero. For older women who have trouble conceiving, there are now options, such as in vitro fertilization and surrogate parenting. Exposure to parents' problematic marriages and painful experience with divorce apparently also tend to make children less enthusiastic about early marriage or even marriage altogether.

Psychotherapy with Adolescents: Different Than with Children and Adults?

Adolescents are a separate animal from either children or adults. The Center's work-ups with teenagers require the therapist to be trigger quick in comprehending the needs and tolerances of the patient. Most commonly, therapists are shocked by the teenager's rapid, even total, shifts in mood and commitments, the teen insistent on getting instant advice and reassurance from the therapist or turning to friends and action to find relief. Also, when the relationship takes, complying with an adolescent's idealized picture of the therapist may run counter to the therapist's belief about desirable therapeutic behavior. The therapist may sense danger in the pleasure that he or she and the patient get when the therapist is elevated to perfection, appropriately finding him- or herself waiting for the other shoe to drop. In contrast, adolescents, especially teenagers, are remarkable in the speed with which they can find the therapy and therapist useless, making it critical that the therapist remain flexible, resilient, and creative in order to make quick recoveries from devaluation.

As with children and in conflict with the description of volatility I have just presented, adolescents are in an excellent position to revise lifelong patterns. They are experimental in their thinking and actions. With a therapist who eventually qualifies, they often can move in impressively productive directions. Therapist beware, however, of competition from friends and fun. The friend and fun factors are omnipresent in work with adolescents. Whether or not they interfere with a smooth therapy experience, they are normal and desirable, provided that they do not get out of hand. Forcefully attempting to block either is a formula for outright war with the adolescent patient and a death knell for the therapy.

Procedure

In preparation for and in conjunction with meetings with the therapist, the teenage subject fills in history and self-assessment symptom-oriented questionnaires, such as the adult or child Neurobehavioral Signs and Symptoms Questionnaire and the Center's History Questionnaire in some cases and the symptom-oriented Symptom Checklist-90. Parents, at times teachers, and therapist fill out complementary forms. The therapist and patient complete the Target Complaint and Goal Attainment Scale questionnaires to track changes in the patient's requirements. The therapist takes progress and process notes.

Self-report inventories including the Beck or Hamilton Depression or Anxiety scales, the BASC for conduct problems, the Behavioral Rating Inventory of Executive Function (BRIEF) to assess neuropsychological functioning, and the Conners' Rating Scales (Short Form) should be completed by the patient, parents, and teachers and, in some cases, by the therapist when appropriate. This task is scheduled at the onset of treatment and again every 6 months with the Rorschach test included at the initial assessment and then approximately every 18 months. Optionally, the Roberts Apperception Test and the Thematic Apperception Test can be added.

As the assessment proceeds, the therapist, with the patient's assent, may decide to make a home visit or hold one or more family sessions. Frequently, it is judicious as well as meaningful to the patient if the therapist and he or she meet on his or her own territory, such as at a fast-food restaurant or on a basketball court.

The timing of testing, collaborative meetings, and sessions is likely to be a particularly sensitive issue for adolescents because of their social schedules. Including them in planning and scheduling is more critical than at any other stage of preadult development.

As in all the Center's cases, the entire battery of psychological tests is again scheduled a few months before termination. Other assessments and consultations, such as educational or vocational, are engaged as needed.

Elaboration on the Central Predicament in Work with Adolescents: A Case Illustration

In many ways, working with adolescents is trickier than with any other age-group. Typically, the adolescent wants parents out of the picture, insisting on his or her ability and right to conduct his or her own life. Nonetheless, as already stated, adolescents, at least in this culture, usually are not financially or emotionally independent, nor, especially prior to age 16 or 17, are they likely to be capable of making sound, safe judgments. So what to do when your patient insists that you keep his or her parents out of the therapy loop? What happens when you know that the parents will work against the interests of that adolescent if you are not in regular contact with them or that regular contact is required since their teenager puts him- or herself in dangerous situations? One caveat. To carry out the procedure I describe, you need to be technically facile, engaging with both the teenager and parents evenly so that in the end the parents and the adolescent get most of what they require from the therapy. I will say one more word about this therapeutic dilemma here and then elaborate on it as part of the description of my work with Ken.

First, it is mandatory to be judicious about what you say to the teenager but also essential that the adolescent be willing and able to keep your more incisive comments about his or her parents' behavior between the two of you. Be aware that even in relationships with adolescents who seem secure and comfortable, adolescent loyalty can turn on a dime. Also, adolescents frequently find themselves becoming disenchanted with a previously idealized therapist and look for reasons to exit therapy. On the other hand, recall that, more than with any other age-group, adolescents tend to insist on openness and authenticity and can develop impressive loyalty when they come to trust a therapist. Even more complicated, you as the therapist need to absolutely trust that the adolescent's parents are committed to the therapy and understand that much of what you and they talk about needs to remain between the three of you. Strategizing with the adolescent while you are in league with his or her parents is not just admissible but often required as well. With maturity and progress, however, the parents increasingly drop out of the picture.

Ken provides a good illustration of many of these principles. Ken, at age 16, was failing all his classes. His mother described him on the phone as surly, possibly drug using. He had lost the right to use his cell phone, and his computer had been removed from his room. His mother, an admirable critical care nurse, did little more than yell at him about doing his work. His father, who drank too much and was mainly ineffectual, supported the mother. As a park ranger, he owned and brandished his law enforcement equipment and skills, threatening mild violence toward Ken and his allegedly no-good friends if Ken remained in violation of family rules. When I saw Ken for the first time, I was certain I had made a mistake taking him on. He greeted me in the waiting room with a grunt from underneath his hooded sweatshirt, which at the time was pulled over his head.

No question. I had a druggie on my hands.

Then Ken began to talk. Shockingly, he was mild. His words were carefully chosen and remarkably sophisticated for a guy who looked like he was straight out of "the hood." The next shock was when the copy of *The Economist* he was reading fell out of his sweatshirt.

So I asked him, "What the hell is this all about?" Wasn't he the loser I had "heard only bad things about?" "What, Ken, is the real story?"

Ken was never very animated, just sparklingly intelligent. He mainly answered my questions, rarely initiating conversation. However, he was always very cooperative. Ken's response was that he intended to pass all his courses next semester, a claim that proved baseless. He insisted that the real problem was that his parents wouldn't let him have any of his vital possessions, including his cell phone, and that they attempted to regulate and patrol him like a prisoner of war.

"Okay, Ken if you want a reprieve, you will have to work closely with me. We will need to meet with your parents in a week or so and again every so often thereafter. You will have to do your best to stop being so surly and actually try in school. You obviously are bright, if not in some ways brilliant, and we need to prove that to you and your parents. Hence the need for at least cognitive testing. How about it?" Note that Ken was clear with me that he did not use drugs and had a goal he felt was more important than school: to achieve the Eagle rank in the Boy Scouts, an organization with which his father was also deeply involved.

So, as is often the case with adolescents, I became a critical advocate for Ken with his parents and the source of good advice. This "real person" role is typical in work with adolescents, who generally do not want to be either dependent on an adult or infantilized. Progressively, they need to prove to themselves and the world that they are capable, autonomous human beings. This requirement lasts all through therapy.

With Ken, I was honest in my agreement that his parents were opaque to his virtues, only seeing and magnifying his failures. With Ken's parents, I openly shared my experiences and impressions of Ken, calling them and leaving a message after every other session with Ken. Both Ken and his parents kept the faith, and both were satisfied.

Adolescent work and therefore the adolescent work-up, then, differ from those with adults and even children. In the beginning, the patient is often there against his or her will and is subject to massive yet normal mood shifts, making the therapy relevant on one day and an anathema on the next. To elaborate on points made earlier, the therapist is almost always in competition with the adolescent's friends for who will share the teenager's confidences, a fact that inevitably creates a therapeutic split. This reality often necessitates that the therapist become creditable not only to the parents and adolescent but also to the patient's friends. With adolescents, the therapist cannot expect the same kind of commitment to thoroughness and completion that he or she has come to associate with adults. Therapy with adolescents is necessarily episodic in that it may start and stop in accordance with the teenager's whims and moods. It is less likely that an adolescent will see the need for testing and be as tolerant of it as an adult might, and he or she may simply need to be forced to do it. Involvement in the psychotherapy by a willing adolescent patient is often more heartfelt than it is with children but not equivalent to what would be expected from an adult. Nonetheless, the adolescent's engagement is likely to vacillate between intense interest and profound disaffection.

Before ending this section, I again want to describe the adolescent therapist's main dilemma. Typically—and certainly characterizing my work with Ken—the therapist of an adolescent is in the paradoxical position of being the patient's advocate while at the same time, if he or she is smart, being in what is often a semisecret alliance with the parents. This alliance at times requires the therapist to privately breach the patient's confidentiality. In part, the therapist needs judiciously to engage in this balancing act since teenagers typically take risks that may put them in jeopardy. They are trying their new wings and have not yet developed adult-level judgment about life. A subtle example of this kind of behavior is Ken's reckless disregard for his schoolwork. He never did his homework, yet he believed with conviction that he would graduate with his classmates and get into a good college. By the way, testing revealed that Ken was as bright as I thought, with one exception. His verbal intelligence was in the superior range, while nonverbal measures found him relatively lacking. This discovery suggested that while he could master intellectual concepts like a wizard, he had a much harder time grasping information about life requirements and comprehending the gravity of other peoples' requirements for him, a discrepancy that was reinforced by his adolescent preference for action and immediate satisfaction.

Our Patients

So now that we have covered diagnosis and monitoring of progress across the diagnostic and developmental spectrum, who are the Center's patients anyway, and how do they know about us? How typical are the group of patients around whom the Center's procedures have been developed? What gives us the right to claim that these procedure are likely to appeal to therapists in office-based practices (Morrow-Bradley & Elliot, 1986)? In the next chapter, I describe how we deliver our services through the Center, and then in chapter 8, I profile our patients.

Appendix

I. Assessment and Monitoring Procedure for Children and Adolescents: Early in course of the assessment the therapist, parents, and, if possible, the patient complete the Target Complaint and Goal Attainment Scale questionnaires. As soon as possible after the start of therapy a psychologist-assessor administers the following assessment instruments: (1) The parents, with the help of the child if feasible, fill out the Child Neurobehavioral History Questionnaire. Self-report inventories are completed, including the BASC for conduct problems and the BRIEF to assess neuropsychological functioning. The Minnesota Multiphasic Personality Inventory can be used as an alternative for evaluating adolescents. The Conners' Ratings Scales are also completed by patient, parents, and teachers. (2) The psychologist-assessor administers the Thematic Apperception (the Roberts Apperception Test or the Children's Apperception Test can be substituted), the Rorschach Test, and the Wechsler Intelligence Scale for Children or for convenience and if appropriate the Wechsler Abbreviated Scale of Intelligence. (3) Other assessment instruments are used as needed.

Each data-gathering and feedback meeting with the psychologist-assessor is conducted collaboratively between him- or herself, the parents, and the therapist, with the psychologist-assessor providing useful consultative input to all. The child or adolescent also attends these meetings when it is clinically appropriate. Two related but separate collaborations are involved in this procedure: the collaboration between the therapist and patient and that involving the psychologist-assessor with the therapist and patient, individually and together.

Ideally, every 6 months the psychologist-assessor (see later in this appendix) returns to make a clinical assessment and to readminister an abbreviated testing battery. The full battery is repeated at approximately 18-month intervals and a few months prior to the end of treatment. This testing and monitoring schedule is the same as that for adults as described in chapter 5. There is at least one feedback session with the psychologist-assessor after each major assessment. Whether feedback for the 6-month retesting occurs over the phone or in person is optional. Cost may be a consideration.

The original psychologist-assessor remains involved throughout the treatment if possible. A medical examination is requested at the beginning of treatment and every year or two thereafter.

II. Details of the Procedure

A. Summary of the Assessment:

1. The following are the steps in the initial assessment procedure, ongoing assessments, and documentation of change. This process is divided into stages, including the initial meetings with the parents, patient, and, as indicated, meetings and phone calls with teachers and caretakers; the clinical assessment by the therapist in collaboration with the parents leading to a preliminary diagnostic formulation; the clinical consultation and testing by the psychologist-assessor; the creation and discussion of a treatment plan that may or may not involve psychotherapy; referral as appropriate; and follow-up. Additional self-report inventories along with appropriate psychological or neuropsychological tests may be completed when specific syndromes such as behavioral problems, attention deficit disorder, depression, or anxiety are at issue. For example, when there are attentional issues that need to be clarified, the BASC and the Conners' self-assessment inventories as well as the Conners' Continuous Performance Test, among others, may add substantially to the power of the assessment. The testing process concludes with one or more collaboratively conducted feedback meetings with the psychologist-assessor. To track the patient's progress symptomatically and in terms of his or her goals, the parents, therapist, and, when possible, child or adolescent complete the Goal Attainment Scale and Target Symptom questionnaires on a biweekly or monthly basis.

Other needed consultations may be added.

B. Breakdown of Assessment and Treatment.

a. Screening call, information to be recorded:
Referral source
Face data

Reasons for referral (who is the informant?)
Fee (discussed? with whom?)
(time: 30 minutes)

b. Materials given or sent to patient and parents:
Fee agreement
Face sheet containing orienting information
Center personal data and history organizers. Added may be other history and self-report inventories addressing specific problems, such as attention deficit disorder or depression.
Permissions (sent? to whom?)

c. Initial meeting (75 to 90 minutes): Often this is simply a screening meeting for parents. Its purpose is for the parents and therapist to form their initial impressions of one another and begin to plan the evaluation. The parents' questions about the evaluation and treatment process, including what it can promise, need to be addressed. Frequently, parents will also want information about the therapist's credentials, theoretical orientation, and personal background. The child or adolescent is usually excluded from this meeting.

The therapist and parents begin to use the Target Complaint and Goal Attainment Scale questionnaires and any other appropriate self-report inventory.

d. Collection of Background Information: The therapist reviews records, including past testing reports and Center history forms (time: usually 30 to 60 minutes). The therapist begins to contact collateral sources of information either by phone or in person. Included are others who have had close contact with or evaluated the patient, including tutors, nannies, teachers, medical doctors, family members, and others. (time: undetermined; usually 1–2 hours)

e. Evaluation, sessions 2 to 5:

Included are the initial meeting(s) with parents, then two to four meetings with the child plus possible home and school visits. At the end, there is a wrap-up session in which a treatment plan and tentative recommendations are collaboratively processed by the parents and therapist. The treatment plan, after it is arrived at, is revised periodically in collaboration with the parents and, if possible, the patient.

f. Possible home and school visit(s)
(time: two to four 75- to 90-minute sessions, plus additional time speaking or meeting with parents and informants; add time required for home and school visits)

g. Treatment according to the arrived-at recommendations follows the assessment period.

If psychotherapy is required, the treatment type is chosen thoughtfully. Possibilities range from interpersonal dynamic psychotherapy or cognitive-behavioral therapy to group therapy. Parental guidance with or without accompanying psychotherapy is likely to be required for work with both children and adolescents. Meetings between the therapist and parents as well as consultations with teachers and sometimes tutors are always part of a treatment plan with children and often for adolescents. Family meetings and at times family therapy may be arranged, usually collateral to individual therapy but at times replacing it. Alternatively or simultaneously, the patient might be referred for tutoring, speech therapy, vocational counseling (if he or she is an adolescent), or any other type of appropriate help. "Environmental engineering" involving a liaison between the therapist and parents may be required. A decision about the therapist's involvement in a legal process may also be at issue. The outcome of the Center assessment may be referral to another professional or a specialist in a needed area.

CHAPTER SEVEN

Delivery of Services: The Center for Collaborative Psychology and Psychiatry

It is through the Center for Collaborative Psychology and Psychiatry that we reach others. Here we apply our methods and do our clinical work, including treatment and referral. We also train therapists to use our model, and we collaborate with other professionals and organizations.

We are acutely aware of the speed with which new technology, especially of a biological nature, is being introduced into our field and the virtual impossibility of any one of us remaining proficient in all areas, hence the diversity we attempt to create among the Center's associates (see chapter 1). Nonetheless, we strive to remain aware of cutting-edge information and technology, including psychological and neuropsychological assessment techniques, and research on the most effective methods of treatment, including medical and pharmacological therapies. Lest this claim seem boastful, think of how you might feel if your medical doctor missed a critical diagnosis or failed to recommend a treatment because he or she was unaware of it or failed to consult with other doctors who were.

In addition to the Center's associates, we make referrals to professionals whose style and competence are well known to us, maintaining an up-to-date list of these people. And, perhaps most important, we have available to us the brainpower and vast experience of the patients we treat. They are engaged as true collaborators and continually surprise us and themselves with how much they know and can contribute to sustaining effective psychotherapy and bringing their lives forward.

Finally, as mentioned in chapter 1, we also collaborate regularly with other centers dedicated to ends similar to our own.

Training of Others in Our Model

Training people to join the professionals with whom we work closely is central to maintaining our vitality. This training occurs in biweekly consultation groups where we get to know and share in the work of the participants and through the seminars we conduct. In addition to training people with whom we can work, we want to create a community of like-minded professionals who can work and grow together.

The Project

Our desire is to create an especially efficient and effective approach to doing and delivering psychotherapy, one that any psychotherapist can readily use for his or her practice. Maintaining this aim requires that we organize our clinical data with a self-monitoring, clinical research goal in mind. For our most objective data, we regularly conduct the Center's testing procedures described in chapters 5 and 6. The results of these assessments are evaluated together with ongoing narrative records from the therapists' notes and self-report inventories, including the Target Complaint and Goal Attainment Scale questionnaires, which we have the patient and therapist fill out every 2 to 4 weeks.

Statistically, we plan to derive effect sizes using data from our psychological and neuropsychological assessments and follow-ups. In this way, we should be able to document how well our patients benefit from our psychotherapies. We should then be able to compare our findings with published data on effect size from studies of psychotherapy. In making this statement, I am acutely aware that as a therapy evolves, its parameters, such as length of sessions and the assessment instruments used, may and often do need to change, hence the imperfect nature of our data. To remain true to our clinical responsibilities, we need to go along with these changes as they occur and confirm their value collaboratively with the patient as well as monitor their utility through reassessment.

What We Offer

In chapters 5 and 6, I described how we at the Center evaluate and follow patients. In addition to providing a medical history and agreeing to obtain a physical examination, every patient needs to consent to an initial battery of psychological or neuropsychological tests and then to regular follow-up using these and other psychometric measures. The timing of this testing is flexible, however, and is a function of the clinical requirements operative in the treatment at the time. The costs need also to be kept reasonable enough so that they are not a deterrent to the patient's ongoing commitment to the evaluation and treatment.

It is necessary that collaboration be maintained between the therapist, the patient, the parents (if the patient is a child or an adolescent), and the psychologist-assessor. As part of the testing and retesting procedure, the patient or parents as well as the therapist provide the psychologist-assessor with a list of questions and comments they would like addressed. These lists are formulated by the therapist and patient or parents independently. The questions and comments need to be straightforward, whether intended to provide the psychologist-assessor with input about the patient's problems or express grievances about the therapy. Both the patient and the therapist see these questions and comments once they are recorded, anticipating that the psychologist-assessor will address them through testing and clinical feedback.

At the end of the formal assessment, the results of the testing are first presented verbally to the therapist and patient so that there is an opportunity for everyone concerned to sift through the psychologist-assessor's findings prior to their being fixed in a report. The psychologist-assessor also has the novel role of proposing and potentially executing remedial strategies complementing the psychotherapy. Generally, these measures include neuropsychological and cognitive-behavioral training in areas where the patient has a deficit. Examples of problem areas particularly amenable to remediation of this sort include difficulties with attention and organization. As a basic requirement for carrying out this ancillary function, the psychologist-assessor has the responsibility of coordinating his or her work with the therapist so as not to duplicate or undermine his or her role.

The psychologist-assessor is also available to work methodically and collaboratively with the patient and, if relevant, his or her parents to assimilate the meaning and implications of his or her testing. Stephen Finn, Ph.D., and Constance Fischer, Ph.D., have recast feedback about assessment and even the experience of the assessment itself so that these have a therapeutic function. They call this technique "therapeutic assessment" (Finn & Fischer, 1997; Fischer, 1994, 2000). At the Center, we have extended these principles, with the psychologist-assessor available to provide regular input to the therapy when it flags or falters (Engelman & Frankel, 2002).

The Reluctance of Therapists to Use the Center's Model

It is unusual for psychotherapists to formally monitor their patients and especially for them to routinely use psychological and neuropsychological testing as part of their diagnostic procedure for adults. Yet doing both makes so much sense, especially if the testing can be made affordable and enhances rather than disrupts the flow of the therapy. Recall my argument from chapter 1 about the need for therapists to augment their credibility by becoming more accountable for the results of their work. To repeat, we as psychotherapists stand out among medical professionals in our seeming disinterest in formally documenting the extent and durability of our patients' progress. It is not that psychotherapists as a professional group are against doing this, it is just that we usually don't.

As a psychotherapist who would have invoked time-worn arguments about risks to the sanctity of the therapist–patient bond of involving a third party, in our case a psychologist-assessor, I now stand firm as a convert to the principle. In the more than 80 cases we have done at the Center (most carried out for well over a year), we have rarely encountered an instance where the patient or parents eventually did not see the testing as a boon to the treatment. When therapist and patient value what they have built together, apparently there is little chance that their work will be diluted by the involvement of a psychologist-assessor. In our experience, the overwhelming probability is that the psychologist-assessor will bolster the treatment by the technical assistance that he or she provides.

As illustrated in following example, the idea of testing and collaboration may be met with distrust by therapists. Introducing these measures may be viewed by the therapist as unnecessary or inconvenient, potentially crimping his or her therapeutic spontaneity. However, while understandable, my impression is that these concerns are often less straightforward than they seem and may be contaminated by the therapist's unwitting need to retain authority and control events in the treatment.

Training Others in Collaborative Assessment and Treatment

Dr. H. is an experienced child psychologist. She was invited to become a Center associate because of our respect for her clinical capability. Contrary to our expectations, the experience was painful for everyone involved. The association misfired with Dr. H's initial Center case, Teddy, a 7-year-old boy both of whose parents were university professors.

The problem apparently started when Dr. H. failed to inform Teddy's parents about the Center's requirement that the parents and therapist maintain a collaborative liaison with the psychologist-assessor so the testing could be experienced as an integral part of the treatment. Instead, Dr. H. insisted that all communication with Teddy's parents occur through her, allegedly to "preserve the integrity of the psychotherapy process." As a result of this failure to comprehend the meaning of the Center's collaborative assessment model, Teddy's parents were led to picture a process where their son would be tested, the tests scored, and the results communicated by report with no or little intervening communication with the psychologist-assessor.

The parents, because of their belief in their son's limitless intelligence, expected to discover that Teddy's problems were circumscribed and could be fixed by a formula. Unfortunately, they couldn't have been more misguided. Contrary to their expectations, testing revealed that Teddy's intelligence was in the average range and that his ability to learn verbally significantly outstripped his almost handicapped nonverbal capability.

Not surprisingly, on receiving the psychologist-assessor's report, the parents were mortified. They immediately blamed the psychologist-assessor for doing an inadequate job. At this point, in spite of her generally good intentions, Dr. H. was in a serious bind. If she sided with the psychologist-assessor, she would also be seen as misguided and technically incompetent, and she would lose the patient.

So what went wrong? Where in this chain of events did Dr. H.'s failure to understand or accept the Center's collaborative assessment model spoil the possibility that the evaluation could succeed? Our retrospective opinion is that Dr. H. was never willing to commit herself to the collaborative assessment model in the first place. Teddy was her patient and she his doctor. According to her conventional view of psychotherapy, she was responsible for Teddy's welfare and would single-handedly bring him through his troubles. Dr. H.'s training and orientation fated this assessment to fail from the beginning. It determined that Teddy's parents would inadvertently arrange for the perpetuation of their illusion and ultimately its consolidation into a fixed belief that they were being victimized by the assessment.

In contrast, had they understood how the Center's collaborative assessment model works, had they and Dr. H. formulated testing questions and opinions in writing prior to the assessment, the need for damage control might have been apparent from the beginning. They actually had been told that this step was a mandatory part of the assessment process but never complied with it. In contrast, a Center-trained therapist most likely would have taken the Center's protocol more seriously and put a stop to the assessment process until everyone involved understood the risks of discovering that Teddy was learning impaired. Data would have slowly emerged, giving the parents the opportunity to acclimate to the unpleasant news they were to receive. As important, they might also have given the psychologist-assessor ample opportunity to help them not only assimilate the psychologist-assessor's findings but also devise remediation strategies with them.

The essential point is that collaboration does not come naturally to many psychotherapists. They tend to practice independently, and training therapists to work collaboratively within the Center's model will need to be a major focus of our attention. As mentioned in chapter 1, it is of interest that in a small study involving time-limited dynamic psychotherapy, Henry, Schacht, Strupp, Butler, and Binder (1993) found that therapists who had less prior supervision and experience were more flexible than those who were more seasoned. This finding led the authors to recommend that competent but relatively less experienced therapists, those less vulnerable to negative effects of training, be selected when new treatments are being offered and taught. Consistent with this finding, we have learned how important versatility and the ability to use good common sense when making clinical decisions are in choosing and training a Center therapist.

This finding notwithstanding, the preponderance of research on the relationship between therapy outcome and therapist competence suggests "that greater competence is related to better outcome . . . though the specific competencies that create this association probably require further elaboration" (Roth & Fonagy, 2005, p. 460). Making the association a bit more intuitive is the observation that "more competent therapists are able to deviate appropriately from technical recommendations with more difficult patients" (Rounsaville et al., 1988). However, as our experience with Dr. H. and the Henry et al. article underscores, level of training and clinical flexibility may not always be correlated.

One implication of these findings for our goals at the Center is that providing a new and better service to patients and colleagues can encounter significant resistance if a therapist's adherence to the model in which he or she was trained and is familiar is fervent (Luborsky et al., 1999). The impediment to progress posed by these kinds of inflexible attitudes cannot be overstated. Measures designed to bring psychotherapists of this sort to a more progressive stance may require a personal paradigm shift. These therapists would need to appreciate the influence of habit and subjectivity on a therapist's convictions and behavior and recognize how personalized and arbitrary their own assumptions about how a therapy should be conducted can be. Most difficult, they would have to shift their own thinking and behavior accordingly.

Our Own Reluctance to Use Center Procedure and Its Consequences

It is not only others who are reluctant to introduce formal procedures into their psychotherapies. I am no different, at times overlooking my failure to engage a psychologist-assessor and integrate his or her testing into my work. My reasons for this neglect are probably similar to those of the average practitioner who instinctively feels that introducing another major player into an already complicated therapy will be inconvenient, confusing, and disruptive.

Usually added are concerns about the integrity of the therapist–patient relationship being violated. There is also the real possibility that the assessor may be temporarily idealized by the patient and that the two could conspire, inadvertently, to undermine the therapy by providing what the patient perceives as an escape route from its rigors.

Ernesto is a 29-year-old unmarried man. He has a master's degree in organizational psychology and currently works in his mother's family's very successful business consulting with mining companies in South America.

When he first came to me at age 7, Ernesto was a land mine. He would fly into rages with almost no provocation. One day, for example, he complained that that his foot hurt. I took the liberty of palpating the allegedly painful area. Ernesto's screaming must have alarmed everyone for miles around. He had suddenly been attacked, and I did it. Our friendly relationship was gone for that day.

I managed this episode as I did all others from then and for several years thereafter. I remained calm and treated it as a hysterical outburst. We never usefully talked about these rages even though years later he acknowledged that they indeed were a problem of his.

I knew it. Ernesto was insufferably spoiled and self-centered. For years, his egocentricity was limitless, free of reflection. It didn't matter how old he was—that piece never changed. And it cost him. He was thrown out of an excellent local boarding school after his second year for not keeping up with the work. It was his arrogance, his lack of concern with usual requirements, that got him. The same thing almost happened after his first year at college.

But I remained assiduously, almost fervently, committed to Ernesto. My powerful involvement grew from what I knew about his experience being the family pariah. Ernesto had been singled out, especially by his father, as the incarnation of evil. He was unrelenting, treating him in a way that can be described only as abusive. If he moved to the right, it was because he wanted to get away with something. If he moved to the left, the father was sure

Ernesto had committed a minor crime. Ernesto's mother, a more reasonable but weak character, simply went along with her husband.

Oddly enough, even though I often attracted their distrust, Ernesto's parents were thoroughly committed to his being in psychotherapy with me and remained so over years of intermittent treatment. I met with them periodically, with Ernesto both expressing his contempt for them and raising no objections about my working collaterally with them. Ernesto knew that I was his advocate and that his parents listened dutifully to what I had to say. Most important for this illustration is the extent to which I gave Ernesto the benefit of the doubt. I was clear that he was thoroughly pigheaded, probably narcissistic, and certainly arrogant. Nonetheless, I managed to see him as a promising human being, potentially sensitive, and very possibly smart. I was also sold on his almost fanatical insistence on ethical behavior for himself and others. I believed that this focus was as an outgrowth of his own experience of injustice within his family. In fact, I made that opinion quite clear to him, labeling it as a residue of the traumatic aspect of his childhood. What I minimized was its self-righteous character. Everyone needed to conform to Ernesto's expectations. If they didn't, there was hell to pay.

In short, with Ernesto, I took on the role of a benign parent who fervently believed in his son. As such, I could minimize his insufferable arrogance and survive his rages unaffected. The fact that I did not face the music about Ernesto and felt so convinced that I was on target is the reason for presenting this illustration.

What did change for Ernesto during high school was the moderation of his effete view of social acceptability. From this time, he began to see value in others who he had earlier seen as his inferiors. Also, in the third year of high school, he began to develop friendships for the first time and tended to keep some of these in spite of his quickness to judge and his susceptibility to rages when he felt misunderstood. Unchanged was his unrelenting contempt for people he believed were his intellectual inferiors, especially his mother and father.

For the first time, during the second half of college, Ernesto began to read assiduously, mainly about psychology, and within 6 months he began to turn in homework, presumably because he had found a subject that fascinated him. After graduation, he applied to doctorate-level psychology programs, finding it hard to comprehend how each one could turn him down. His self-importance prevented him from accepting their judgment as valid. He concluded self-righteously that there must be something inconsequential impeding his admission and that he would try again sometime later. Previously, his incessant excuse making as a student and in his life in general caused others—and always his parents—to dismiss his ideas out of hand. Nonetheless, Ernesto earned a master's degree from a credible school and reentered therapy with me claiming that he wanted to know as much as possible about where his rages came from.

Ernesto became much more tolerable to be with at about age 26 after he discovered Bikram yoga. Here was a place for Ernesto to shine as a contortionist. He was athletic, lithe, and supple; he liked the philosophy supporting Bikram yoga and eventually decided to become a part-time teacher. Here was another mark of superiority in the making. It was just that the Bikram yoga instructors didn't see it that way. Apparently, they did not feel he was qualified to become an instructor. He was forced to give up his quest to become a Bikram yoga master, dissolving into a burst of irritation about how he found them inadequate, and had decided to simply continue a meditation practice on his own.

But Bikram yoga did help. Ordinarily, Ernesto was able now to calm himself and detach from his emotions, an impressive "therapeutic" result.

And I kept directing Ernesto. I felt clear that he was wiser and even smarter than his parents. I insisted that, for him, justice should involve not letting his two brothers run away with the mother's family fortune as his mother's brothers had done with his mother. I was not shy about suggesting that the way for him to right past wrongs might well be to reinstate himself into the family and even join the mother's family business.

The problem is that I believed this outcome unlikely. Ernesto's father was so hateful toward him that his diabolic view of his alleged malevolence seemed almost delusional. Each time I listened to his father's diatribe against Ernesto, I felt enraged, even agitated, and thoroughly pessimistic about Ernesto's chances of reliably reinstating himself within his family.

However, with my help, Ernesto progressively discovered exactly what to do. Compromising his over-strong ethical system he ostensibly joined with his mother who had conditionally reentered the famly business. To survive and, indeed, to succeed, he took direction from me at each hairpin turn. After about a year of employment by his mother's family, Ernesto began to earn the mother's and her family's respect for his competence and even his reliability. In fact, after a year and a half, his previously critical and controlling mother began to give him full responsibility for managing a small family-owned enterprise.

This shift in his mother's attitude triggered Ernesto's desire to establish more independence in his role in the mother's family business. I understood, yet I was alarmed. An abrupt change of direction could be dangerous for Ernesto, again inviting his parents to distrust his motivations. I counseled him that before acting, he might want some guarantee that if his parents reversed field and again became devaluing, as his grandfather had done with his mother, he should have something to sustain himself financially. I suggested that he begin a campaign to have his mother put some assets that Ernesto already regarded as his own in Ernesto's name.

Along with these developments, Ernesto handled his mother's and her family's incessant criticisms at work primarily by invoking meditative self-control. While this equanimity was forced, his professional competence was increasingly recognized by his mother and her family members with whom Ernesto worked. At this point, Ernesto's father for the most part dropped his hypercritical stance with Ernesto. Although his tirades continued, for the first time in Ernesto's life, they were muted by his mother, who argued with her husband that Ernesto's performance had become laudable.

Appropriately, at this point, Ernesto suggested that our work should be about over. Coordinately, a few months earlier, Ernesto's father, in frustration I think, wondered whether Ernesto should be finishing his treatment with me. He thought that Ernesto's seeing someone different might overcome what he alleged was my tendency not to comprehend Ernesto's inherent malevolence. Admittedly, I simply dispensed with this suggestion as yet another attempt by the father to condemn his son.

The problems I perceived with Ernesto's later suggestion that we finish treatment, however, are intriguing. Ernesto had a distinct tendency to overestimate himself. While he felt ready, even anxious, to spend his trust fund money on his own investments, his mother and those in whom she confided thought he needed at least another year of business experience before he even began to invest it. From what I knew about the limitations of Ernesto's experience in business, I agreed, assuming that Ernesto could easily be taken in by a slick businessmen who made him feel important.

Also, Ernesto's father's naysaying always echoed in the background. More powerfully, he continued to use every opportunity with his wife to cut Ernesto out of the business, acting as if Ernesto could be trouble for his mother. In spite of Ernesto's mother's moderation, she never gained full faith in Ernesto's intentions or even his competence.

With his father ever ready to see his faults and forget his impressive professional and personal progress and his mother's accurate judgment of how his overconfidence might distort Ernesto's choices of investments and partners, Ernesto was probably more personally dependent on my guidance and my intervention with his parents than he wanted to admit. Here I am thinking about guidance as having a therapeutic as well as an interpersonal function, acquainting Ernesto with his latent grandiosity and eventually helping him to contain it. Also, acknowledging my point of view as meaningful could theoretically continue to move Ernesto from a world in which the only subjective experiences of importance were his own to one in which others had a place.

Should I then not have been shocked when Ernesto abruptly greeted me one Monday with "I want you to be clear I'm not coming back"? "You helped me a lot for a long time but for the past year, maybe several years, our relationship has been a problem for me. Our conversations force me to focus on my parents' limitations, re-create the reasons for my rages. I've already written them off and don't want to be reminded of their deficiencies. Since you won't hear me, I'll have to take things into my own hands and end today. I'll be in touch after a couple of months. I can confide in my friends. or maybe I'll find another therapist to talk with." The litany continued. His tone became even more accusing. "You let me down by not making a concrete plan at each point in our work like other therapists do, not even taking notes regularly."

"But what makes you think we didn't make plans and that I didn't take notes?" I retorted, feeling misunderstood. As if he hadn't heard me, he cited his friends' therapists who he claimed were "concrete and clear."

Ernesto looked like he could murder me. I recognized that look from past misunderstandings. It was an angry, frightening scowl that screamed violence. At that moment, while being decimated by his stare, I recalled, this time viscerally, his father's incessantly hateful tirades involving Ernesto and, before that, the appalling abuse his mother experienced from her own father and then her brothers who followed suit.

I stood my ground. "Ernesto, I believe we need at least two more meetings. At minimum, we haven't finished reviewing the consequences of your having been so unappreciated by your parents and how that impacts your life now."

Invoking a time frame like his mother's, I privately believed we needed at least a year more to complete our work. In my case, the specific agenda was to more rigorously review Ernesto's past with him and vigorously flush out his traumatic experience as the family pariah. I felt protective, unwilling to take his self-assurance at face value. Sadly, however, all I thought I could bargain for were two sessions, hoping they would provide an opening for Ernesto to cool down and reconsider his actions. While I agreed with his claim that independence from his parents and me were the next steps, I believed he was talking himself into believing that he was there already.

"I know," he retorted, "but you were supposed to do that during the past few months." Then, moment by moment, he got even more angry and stubborn, finally stalking out of my office at the last moment of our meeting.

Before he left, however, he stated that my proper place in his future was only in my work with his parents. He held firm to that view, even as I made it clear that my condition for continuing to work with his parents was that he be willing to collaborate with me, keep me informed, and repeatedly make his needs clear to me. And it hurt. In spite of myself, I couldn't help thinking, "Didn't I rescue Ernesto from certain destruction and tenderly nurture him to the point where he could be a fully integrated family member and inherit the share of the family fortune he was due? Didn't I, for years, put myself out on a limb, risking the parents' censure?"

A few days later, after not hearing from him, I left a message. "You know that I've had a meeting for next week scheduled with your father, so I'll just go ahead with it as if everything is normal. You can take your time. I hope you will get in touch with me. Apart from wanting to better understand what has happened between us, I value our relationship and hope we can salvage what is good about it. That aside, I cannot continue to work with your parents without your full assent and support. So, unless you are willing to join me in any future work with them, there can be no more meetings with them beyond that one."

We talked several times during the next few months but always about my discussions with his parents. Ernesto remained icy and rageful when I attempted to reintroduce that subject. He did agree, however, to speak with me again after returning from an impending trip to Peru. His plan was to teach business psychology methods to indigenous people, who in his eyes were unjustly trapped by their pitiful circumstances.

So what happened to my rock-solid bond with Ernesto?

Is it possible that the Ernesto I encountered face-to-face, fist-to-fist, in that last formal therapy session was the "real" Ernesto? Could this be the diabolical person who had always frightened his father? Perhaps I was suffering from an impairment of memory and clinical judgment, forgetting what I had known for years about Ernesto's temperamental failings, his being so easily provoked to anger and critical judgment. Had I underestimated the psychological consequences of the abuse he had constantly experienced, believing that I was immune from becoming the target of his vindictive rage? Might the delusion have been mine rather than his father's, based on my need to believe in Ernesto's unlimited potential and my seemingly endless ability to bring it out? Yet those convictions had allowed me to help Ernesto for so many years.

A historical note might help since my experience with my own father has parallels to Ernesto's. While I was not conscious of its influence as I worked with Ernesto, this aspect of my background most likely was instrumental in maintaining my fervent empathy with Ernesto's plight. Originally ambitious to distinguish himself as an educator, my father had been blacklisted by the McCarthy committee in the early 1950s, halting his already impressive advance to prominence. As a result, he became bitter and reclusive, giving up his role as father and committing all his time to earning a Ph.D., which he correctly believed would be his professional redemption. At the same time, I was earning honors in every part of my high school experience and had decided that I might go into science or medicine, following my father's original ambition to go to medical school. My inference is that my father may have felt competition with me and redirected his frustrated disappointment about his own life toward me. The result: incessant censure of my attempts to succeed, framed by vituperative rages similar to those experienced by Ernesto.

I suffered enormously from the role in which my father cast me, and, like Ernesto, I organized my own sense of justice in part around these experiences. I swore to myself that my children would never feel misunderstood in the way I had. In effect, Ernesto was my first child. I simply wanted to focus on his potential, just what my father could not do with me.

Of course, I have been forced by this last chapter of my experience with Ernesto to be more realistic about him. In the end, it looks like Ernesto's father had a good point. His truly paranoid warning system may not have been so inaccurate. And I, hero, Ernesto's savior, have egg on my face.

A potentially more important consideration, as I have thought about and discussed this case with colleagues, is Ernesto's character. An even more likely explanation for Ernesto's suddenly turning on me may have to do with his inheritance. He is about to turn 30, just the time that a sizable trust becomes available to him. He will begin to inherit a great deal of money. I have not wanted to think that his reasons for continuing to work so assiduously with me for so long and then breaking it off abruptly over the past several months could be so venial. Others have suggested this explanation, but for a long time I could not even entertain the possibility that it might be true.

However, when I picture the coldness of Ernesto's dismissal of me and the murderous look on his face during that last meeting, I have had to consider even this ultimately cynical explanation. After all, this is the exact time Ernesto will come into the money I struggled so hard to make sure he received. Ernesto is often carried away with an inflated sense of his self-importance. In his own words, he now believes that he is "a successful businessman." Apparently, he feels that he doesn't need me now, believing that if we continued to work together, I would simply impede him.

The major problem here, then, appears to be my chronic overestimation of Ernesto's depth, my insistence on the authenticity of his good intentions, and my underestimation of his egocentricity. Indeed, his politics reflected a personal code of ethics dramatically more humanitarian than that of his parents. After all, he was going to Peru for 6 weeks this summer to train indigenous people in business psychology. As a qualification, however, he was going under the auspices of a private program that required him to pay a considerable tuition. Nonetheless, this undertaking provided Ernesto with sizable self-aggrandizement. While Ernesto claimed that he believed in this mission powerfully, in many ways I was beginning to conclude that his commitment to the lofty ideals he articulated was based significantly on his desire to be seen as and feel heroic.

There are several general questions that a case like this brings up. How often do we as psychotherapists manifest such shortsightedness? If we frequently do, is it possible that our behavior might temporarily and paradoxically be constructive for the clinical process since it supports our role as the patient's advocate? If, in the short term, oversights of this sort can be clinically advantageous, facilitating a conjunctive process, at what point do they—or did they in Ernesto's case—become limiting, masking or supporting pathology?

And, once again, the moral of this story is clear. Ernesto never was tested or monitored using the Center's procedures. Had he been, the events just recounted might have been averted. Most likely, my misjudgment would have been curbed, and both views of Ernesto, the idealized and hoped for as well as the more objective, would have been available to us to work with. The warnings might have come early and been confirmed by assessment. Notice of Ernesto's deficits would undoubtedly have reoriented me and made me more effective as his therapist.

Follow-up: About 2 weeks after our last session, I had my scheduled visit with Ernesto's father. His mother came along. At their request, I met with the father separately, then spoke with the mother, and then met with them together. Both were feeling some alarm, seeing rising signs of arrogance in Ernesto's part in his conduct at work. His father, as usual, was more vituperative than his mother, believing that Ernesto should be out of the business altogether. One difference was that while Ernesto's father always seemed wildly irrational to me earlier, his picture of Ernesto was beginning to gain credibility in my mind. It was my own experience with Ernesto's unempathic, inflexible, and apparently self-serving behavior that was beginning to create this shift in my perception.

Yes, Ernesto's father had chronically overstated Ernesto's malice, seeing him as a duplicate of his wife's father. His father-in-law had seriously abused his daughter, Ernesto's mother, finally cutting her out of his substantial will and leaving Ernesto's mother's fair share to his sons. Over time, the grandfather's ire evolved into paranoid rage episodes directed at Ernesto's mother. Moreover, the rages were strategically fueled by her sons, in a manner not unlike that of the two evil daughters in the Shakespearean tragedy *King Lear*. This drama, together with an earthquake that destroyed part of the family's home, had exhausted Ernesto's father. To make matters worse, his wife remained slavishly dutiful to her father, causing her to continue to act abusively toward her husband and young son. In fact, because of the family's prominence, the legal case by her brothers to disinherit Ernesto's mother had become a local spectacle, causing havoc in Ernesto's household and especially for his father. As part of this spectacle, the battering that Ernesto's father received from both his father-in-law and his wife, while at first unacknowledged, evolved into ridicule by his wife and even his children.

Ernesto's father's only recourse back then was to pay a secret visit to me to seek help for himself and his son, insisting at first that I have no communication with his wife. His son, Ernesto, was out of hand, rampaging the house and, even at his age, terrorizing everyone. He needed my help with Ernesto and in bringing his wife into line as a mother.

So, finally, I was beginning to appreciate his point of view. His fear that if he confronted his wife too directly she would withdraw even further was realistic. While exaggerated, he expected Ernesto to become diabolical as a repetition of his wife's father's treatment of her and her family. To a point, Ernesto's father had little choice but to favor his daughter and grow evermore frightened that Ernesto had inherited his grandfather's temperament. No one, not even I, accorded his view any validity. We all, in effect, conspired in driving this unsophisticated, reactive man progressively crazy.

And here is where it was left for years. During that time, I restored Ernesto's father to his paternal role, fixed his parents' marriage, and clarified Ernesto's sister's ill will toward him while never, however, appreciating that the father might understand Ernesto better than the rest of us. So, the father, after years of being discounted, was finally making sense to me. Sadly, as a commentary about how limiting a therapist's judgment can be without the benefit of testing and consultation, it had taken me all these years to understand what he knew about all along: the distortion in Ernesto's character.

There is little doubt that psychological testing, especially projective testing early on and serial testing later through Center work-ups, would have exposed the self-serving nature of Ernesto's exaggerated sense of justice. From a young age, his impatience might have started to looked like narcissism in the making or even incipient paranoia, his experience of degradation and even abuse from early childhood being key determinants. With this information, I might have spent more time working in therapy with Ernesto's building self-righteousness rather than primarily supporting his indignation and exhorting his parents to see his alleged hidden goodness and abundant untapped strengths.

Certainly, my impressions and methods had some merit. Ernesto needed all the encouragement he could get from his parents and then from me in substitution for what they couldn't provide. But it was the flip side that I missed: Ernesto's growing rage and malevolence. In this case, my certainty that I understood Ernesto and his family's psychology led me to be self-deceptive enough that my ability to serve him over time was compromised. Indeed, beginning in high school, Ernesto had made remarkable progress both in school and with relationships. For that perhaps I should get some credit. It was the narcissism I missed.

The Future of the Center and the Rest of This Book

While I have emphasized the delivery of services through the Center, as vital to our interests is our training program. As illustrated by Dr. H., it may be difficult for psychotherapists to accept and then practice the collaborative model. There is no doubt that Dr. H. felt friendly to the idea of collaborative treatment. She is a friend and trusted colleague. She never meant to betray me. But she did, contaminating what might have been a successful therapeutic intervention.

However, it is not just our associates who need to abide by the Center's protocol, making sure their own desires and misconceptions do not contaminate their judgment. The case of Ernesto has been instructive for me and my Center colleagues and is personally painful for me to relate. But why should I be any more immune to the ravages of wishful thinking based on my personal preferences and prejudices than any of my peers?

The challenge of how to work most effectively through the Center will require thought, experience, and continual revision. Here we need to grapple with such issues of therapist ambition and distortion and their effect on assessment and treatment. We will have to take on the problem of why therapists resist accountability in their clinical work, including that provided by a psychologist-assessor who serves as a consultant to the therapy. Our ultimate challenge is to establish not only that our methods work but also that they are an improvement on those that therapists ordinarily employ. We need also to confirm that they can and will be used by therapists in their offices.

So, at the Center, our problem is people, how they can aid and confuse. I am talking not just about other people but about ourselves as well. Since we are actors in our own drama, we will always need to seek fresh perspectives. Otherwise, we may be seduced into believing that the truth will reveal itself simply from within the bounds of the well-worn paths we are used to taking, hence the mandate that our work be open to scrutiny and that we never be satisfied with the status quo.

CHAPTER EIGHT

Our Clinical Population: A Pilot Study

Twenty-five patients currently or previously in psychotherapy with me were profiled for this clinical survey according to the following characteristics: age; gender; socioeconomic position, including their ability to afford assessments and treatment provided by the Center for Collaborative Psychology and Psychiatry; diagnosis, including whether a constitutional or developmental component was identified as causing or contributing to their condition; inferred capacity to engage in insight-oriented psychotherapy; motivation for change; and whether they required pharmacotherapy. All these subjects received psychological testing at the onset of treatment. Most entered therapy before the current version of the Center's procedures were complete and before guidelines for our current project were thoroughly formulated. Of this group, 15 had completed psychotherapy when this chapter was written. Five remain in treatment, enabling us to retest them regularly according to current Center procedure, while five of them went only as far as completing a full initial assessment. We have maintained contact with all patients from this group who completed treatment, using a variety of interview, self-report, and, when possible, testing methods to track them.

On beginning treatment, all 25 subjects received a full battery of psychological tests with the addition of neuropsychological testing for seven, leaving 18 who received standard clinical testing only. Our battery included a neuropsychological screening device for adults called the Neuropsychological Impairment Scale and from late childhood throughout adulthood the Wechsler Abbreviated Scale of Intelligence or the Wechsler Intelligence

Scale for Children or the Wechsler Adult Intelligence Scale (WAIS) for assessing cognition. Neuropsychological tests were added as required from the Flexible Neuropsychological Battery. Additional testing during and following treatment was done with 20 of these patients. All patients except 10 were assessed less regularly than is our current practice. The protocols for retesting and follow-up were less strictly followed in this pilot project than is standard for our new patients. Now and in the future, we will have even more complete records of our patients' evolving complaints, response to treatment, and progress through formal testing, self-assessment questionnaires, and the ongoing use of the Target Complaint and Goal Attainment Scale questionnaires. As always, therapist notes will be retained, and when an outside therapist or consultant is involved, he or she will be asked to submit periodic written reports.

Office-Based Practice

The "unclean" character of office treatment leads advocates of empirically supported treatment (EST) to the conclusion that real-world psychotherapy should be conducted according to manualized procedures, especially those for individual diagnostic categories (Westen, Novotny, & Thompson-Brenner, 2004). Westen et al. (2004) offer a corrective to attitudes idealizing the use of ESTs. They contend that manualized treatments are "neither well-validated nor broadly applicable to most disorders" (p. 632). Predicating treatments on research-derived principles represents an oversimplification of psychotherapy as it is actually delivered. The patients whom clinicians most commonly encounter in their offices tend to depart from the clear-cut diagnostic criteria of the *Diagnostic and Statistical Manual of Mental Disorders* (4th ed.; *DSM-IV*). Character pathology, the *DSM-IV* axis II classification of "Personality Disorder," usually plays a part in their clinical presentation. This observation reduces the practical value of many manualized protocols, making them only approximately applicable to office-encountered patients. Repeating a point made in chapters 1 and 2, 40% to 70% of those applying for inclusion in most studies are eliminated as unsuitable because of the complexity of their clinical presentation, and many dropped out before their course of treatment was completed. Further, unlike patients encountered in office-based practice, patients recruited for research studies tend to be followed only for as long as the research protocol requires. Also, the interpersonal or behavioral psychotherapies offered are generally short term and focused, lasting for only weeks to months.

Roth and Fonagy (2005), in their book *What Works for Whom*, challenge the assumption that therapists should uniformly shift to manual-based practice. In effect, they support the previously mentioned critique by Westen et al. (2004) by providing a remarkably detailed account of the current state of research about specific types of psychosocial treatment. In 2002, Fonagy and colleagues published the first edition of another, similar book summarizing current research on treatment for children and adolescents (Fonagy, Target, Cottrell, Phillips, & Kurtz, 2002). In referring to this age-group, they note, like Westen et al., that "most psychosocial treatment studies have not included long-term follow-ups," consist of short-term focused treatments, and fail to adequately cover the range of possible treatments, including pharmacotherapy administered with or separately from the psychotherapy. They add the self-evident observation that "child-treatment occurs during a period of rapid cognitive change, and cognitive development is likely to interact with (and confound) treatment inputs" (p. 31).

Add to these concerns about the limitations of manualized procedures in office-based psychotherapy the dialogues contained in the edited book by Norcross, Beutler, and Levant (2006). Supported are findings such as Wampold's (2001) that most powerful in making psychotherapy work are general "contextual" factors. It of interest that Michael Lambert, the current editor of *Bergin and Garfield's Handbook of Psychotherapy and Behavioral Change* (2004), also treats Wampold's work quite respectfully. In fact, in his own research, Lambert (2007) advocates "monitoring each client's treatment response and making treatment length a function of treatment response and mental health rather than arbitrary or theory-driven limits" (p. 4). Indeed, manualized treatment protocols do have their limitations when applied to office-based patients, and the importance of appropriate responsiveness to the patient at each clinical moment cannot be underestimated. Nonetheless, the argument that each case has its own technical requirements and that, to maximize outcome, specific interventions need to be formulated accordingly squares solidly with my own clinical experience.

Our Two Pilot Projects

We have designed the Center's diagnostic and monitoring procedures so that they can be conveniently and economically used by office-based clinicians to assess their patients and follow their progress. Here is how these procedures were developed during our first two pilot projects (Frankel, 1995), the second being the one described in this chapter. We have currently initiated another clinical study using finalized Center protocols for the initial assessment, monitoring of progress, and follow-up. Also, our record-keeping system has been improved for this project and is more reliable. All three studies were conceived of and developed by myself and Philip Erdberg, Ph.D. Through our experience treating and testing many of the roughly 25 patients in each study, we have evolved our system of assessment and monitoring, tightening it with each new group.

In the study I describe in this chapter, our second clinical study, I collected my data as follows. First, I took careful on-the-spot process notes as I did psychotherapy or psychoanalysis with my patients. I then submitted these records to well-trained and experienced colleagues for appraisal. Without commentary from me, they meticulously reviewed my notes and commentary, making observations about the psychotherapy segment reviewed and noting what information was lacking and what measures would improve outcome. Second, as described earlier, during all of these studies, we have always had a psychologist-assessor as part of the treatment team. Generally, the same psychologist-assessor remained available throughout each treatment and the follow-up period. Feedback came through the psychologist-assessor's clinical impressions, psychological and neuropsychological testing, and formal monitoring of progress. The current undertaking was preceded by another clinically based project I conducted. That study involved 30 patients and was carried out over about 5 years. Now that our pilot studies are complete, we are well into a new, third project using formal Center diagnostic assessment and monitoring procedures.

It was through the first project that Phil and I evolved the notion of the three-person therapy field (Frankel, 1995). We had become convinced of the value of involving a third, independent opinion to counter the subjectivity introduced into the therapy field by both the patient and the therapist. When the input from this third person is tempered by the results of psychological and neuropsychological testing, the perspective offered can be counted on to add another, useful viewpoint for judging the therapy. In *Making Psychotherapy Work: Collaborating Successfully with Your Patient* (Frankel, 2007), I reviewed our survey of study participants to determine how the addition of the psychologist-assessor was regarded by the participants. While at first many of these people were concerned that the psychologist-assessor inclusion would disrupt the privacy of the therapy and worried about the extra costs involved, nearly all participants ultimately found the relatively independent perspective that the psychologist-assessor and testing brought to the treatment reassuring. They typically cited the protection it afforded against the influence of the therapist's and patient's capricious opinions and actions.

In short, almost all participants came to endorse the new procedure as a useful adjunct to what is ordinarily a very subjective process.

The Current Project

Using testing-derived data and clinical impressions, a summary of the breakdown of this current, second pilot study of 25 patients follows.

Descriptive Data

Four patients were children or adolescents: one age 7, and three between 11 and 18 (one in middle school and two in high school). Twenty-one were adults: 11 between 20 and 30 years, three between 30 and 50, and seven over 50.

Twelve participants were males, and 13 were females. All were American born. Two were second-generation Asian American, two second-generation Mexican American, and the rest Caucasian or of mixed heritage. Twelve were professionals or, if children or adolescents, had professionals as parents. The rest had modest but reliable incomes.

Diagnoses

While most of our patients suffered from depression or anxiety and nearly all felt thwarted in some area of his or her life either professionally or in relationships, none was considered to be psychotic. Noteworthy is that 10 out of 25 were judged by history and symptoms to be experiencing a trauma-related psychiatric condition, symptomatically experienced by most of these patients as depression or anxiety.

Asked to categorize their sometimes considerable problems, each would have said that they were having trouble managing some aspect of his or her life. That statement is far less simple than it may sound since rarely if ever did the difficulty, as we came to understand it, fit neatly into a *DSM-IV* diagnostic category. How to categorize a crisply diagnosed patient with an added attentional problem or handicapping dyslexia? How about the few who overused alcohol or marijuana? One successful woman was a chronic manipulator who, in spite of her professional achievements, repeatedly alienated people. How to incorporate that into her bipolar diagnosis?

Supporting our consternation about diagnosing was the fact that so much of what had to be done in each psychotherapy required clinical flexibility and judgment. One patient who was depressed required that the therapist make room for his need for certainty from those he depended on, and another with almost the same presentation needed to learn about the personal and social value of doubt and humility. What to call these two cases diagnostically given their similarities? After all, if a diagnosis is accurate, it should be helpful for planning the treatment, should it not?

Childhood Deprivation and Delayed and Arrested Development

Thirteen of the 25 reported emotional deprivation during childhood or adolescence, most in the form of inadequate parenting. Of these, some deliberately sought a reparenting experience from psychotherapy, looking to the psychotherapist for guidance and nurturing they reported missing during their early years. The others recognized that they had this goal only as treatment progressed. Incidentally, there did not seem to be any correspondence between this patient requirement and their socioeconomic status, current financial resources, or level of education.

In comparison to this first group, whose positive response to support or treatment suggested that the aspects of development at issue were delayed, five others were judged arrested in key areas of their expected, normative development. The compromised capacities at issue were mainly depth and maintenance of relationships and egocentricity versus the capacity for empathy. In effect, those people with a developmental arrest needed to start from scratch and learn personal and interpersonal skills that had been present but dormant in the first, delayed development group.

Capacity to Use Insight

Seventeen (68%), tellingly, were judged to be limited in either their capacity or their motivation to use insight-directed therapy. With guidance and encouragement, however, 13 of these people (52%) were able to make significant changes through therapy in the direction of symptom relief and progress in life. Of this group, five were judged to be distinctly more self-reflective by the time they finished treatment, and one who was 16 years old showed convincing indications that she would develop this capacity. Nonetheless, nine patients wanted an interpretive dimension as part of their psychotherapy, and all patients in the study said that they were interested in gaining some understanding of the cause and nature of their problems.

Patients Who Left Before Completion

Four patients left the Center after the initial assessment and never began treatment. Three were in the child–adolescent category. All three stopped because their parents were satisfied with the assessment only and the burst of progress resulting from it.

Collaboration with Parents or Spouses

In six cases, three of whom were at least in their early 20s, therapist contact with significant others, including parents and spouses, was helpful to the patient. In two other adult cases, including Gary from chapters 3 and 4, the patient was holding his or her parents or a spouse emotionally hostage, for example, by insisting that the person take care of him or her financially or emotionally. In Gary's case, his insistence that he had an incurable psychiatric condition and the complicity of several psychotherapists ensured that this slavish bond to his parents would go unchallenged. Freeing the patient to progress by encouraging significant others to remove themselves emotionally or materially from providing for the patient's care was critical to the success of these treatments.

Use of Medications

Regarding biological interventions, nine (36%) patients required psychotropic medication. Six required sustained treatment with an antidepressant, and one of these patients simultaneously needed a benzodiazapine for anxiety. One required a benzodiazapine to help regulate her intermittent desire to abuse alcohol. One of the patients given an antidepressant also required moderate doses of a mood stabilizer to contain his emotional instability, bordering on bipolarity. One required a benzodiazapine for control of tics. Another needed stimulants to combat attention deficit disorder.

Conditions with a Biological or Temperamental Basis

Eleven (44%) of our patients, including most who required medication, were judged to have some kind of built-in idiosyncrasy, such as impassivity, an attentional disorder, or a hypomanic predisposition. This personality-based factor typically influenced the therapist's style, such as the therapist becoming especially active with inherently passive patients or providing a regulating function for those who were hypomanic and, therefore, impulsive.

Summary and Conclusions: Our Impressions and Their Implications for Center Treatments

Approximately 70% of the patients seen as part of this project were limited in either their ability or their motivation to use insight, about 50% required developmental supplementation with the therapist serving as a parentlike figure, and about 45% seemed temperamentally idiosyncratic, requiring the therapist to adjust his style accordingly. About 40% benefited from medication for at least part of their therapy. It may be surprising that 40% of these patients seemed to have problems associated with earlier trauma, whether or not there had been deprivation in their childhood. Further, even though only about 20% of our adult cases required that the therapist work with significant others in their lives, it was our impression that in those cases the therapist's willingness to provide such adjunctive help was instrumental in creating the interpersonal framework required for therapeutic progress. This part of the treatment can frequently be time limited, provided that the significant other can use the therapist's guidance.

A traditional therapist relying primarily on a patient's capacity to use self-reflection would likely find these impressions discouraging. Yet what else would one expect from a typical practice? After all, these patients represent our (and, I warrant, most office-based therapists') spectrum of patients: a heterogeneous group of frequently talented people who haven't been able to make it well enough on their own. That psychotherapy should consist in part of developmental, pharmacological, and guidance supplementation as well as stylistic readjustment on the part of the therapist is exactly what we would have expected. Thus, the abiding question is, What individualized treatments are required, indeed optimal, for each of these people? Here we get inventive since we have to. Each treatment becomes a complex puzzle to be solved, and the solving can occur only incrementally over time, like any good mystery. As a reminder, the accuracy of each treatment evolves along three therapeutic pathways: (a) collaboration involving therapist and patient by themselves, (b) collaboration between the psychologist-assessor and the therapist and patient individually and jointly, and (c) as a result of the input of repeated assessments done according to the Center's protocol. These are the truing mechanisms that are built into the Center's procedure. In psychotherapy, interpersonal influence is ubiquitous, with information continually exchanged between each of the participants. Much of this activity is unacknowledged, as is the role of the patient's and therapist's intuition and judgment in shaping the treatment.

And the end product. That's the potentially remarkable part. The major and most cogent finding emerging from this work is the unpredictability of the outcome. If the therapy is structured so that it is optimally responsive to the patient's current needs, our repeated experience is that, in addition to amelioration of the presenting problems, potentialities not heretofore appreciated by either the patient or the therapist are likely to emerge, and not necessarily on schedule. The patient discovers interests, emotional and interpersonal capabilities, and talents he or she often hadn't even guessed existed. If the work can be sustained long enough, these discoveries are consolidated into an array of new capabilities and interests, including changes in professional direction, new life patterns including further schooling, expansion and deepening of relationships, marriage, and children. How this happens, especially when it isn't deliberately orchestrated, the "magic" to which I've referred in earlier chapters, is a central focus for our interest. While at times psychotherapy can remain unproductive of change or even be misguided, when it is fine-tuned enough to the patient's needs, it can be a remarkably potent agent of change and discovery.

Returning to the Medical Model

The fact that relative certainty about diagnosis and optimal treatment frequently appears to be so much more elusive in psychotherapy than in general medicine should be no surprise. I understand that this generalization may not hold up under statistical scrutiny and that there is a strong argument for the equivalence of the reliability of the two types of assessments (Meyer et al., 2001). Still, psychotherapists like myself find ourselves acutely aware of the subjectivity and complexity of our clinical work. We in psychiatry and psychology are indeed targeting the soul along with the psychological factors that we can categorize, such as symptoms and personality disorders. The variations in what we encounter and in the creative solutions we can arrive at are extraordinary, and the element of surprise, often surprise on the upside, is ever present.

However, in effect, we psychotherapists are all medical practitioners. We do have the patient's welfare in our hands. The therapist's responsibility to take charge of the therapy, monitor its progress, and include the patient as a full collaborator, while always striving toward objectivity in the clinical work, is never absent.

Brief Case Example: A Typical Center Patient, Benjamin

Benjamin is one of many Center patients. Distinguishing his case is that from the start he was willing to commit to only 1 year of 75-minute once-a-week psychotherapy sessions, later extended to a year and a half. On the other hand, he has been quite cooperative with follow-up since stopping treatment 3 years ago and says he is pleased with the work we did together.

Benjamin is 53 years old. He is a successful accountant in a solo practice. He attended an Ivy League college and has a master's in business administration from a credible graduate school. Benjamin was referred by his wife, an occupational therapist. He has three sons, one of whom graduated from college a year ago.

Benjamin did not come for treatment on his own initiative. Instead, he came at his wife's behest, creating a limitation in our work that we never entirely transcended. His wife was quite concerned about emotional limitations in their relationship. That said, Benjamin had profound respect for his wife and earnestly wanted to understand her dissatisfaction. He did not, however, fully grasp her concerns about their relationship, which characteristically he felt was perfect.

According to his wife, Benjamin also had problems with intimacy reaching beyond their relationship. This contention confused Benjamin since he viewed himself as altruistic and caring. He knew intuitively, however, that she was correct and wanted to understand more about this alleged deficit. At the beginning of treatment and often throughout, Benjamin repeated that he admired his wife and wished to emulate her ability to make and keep close friends. Benjamin claimed that he also had many long-term friends, all, however, male. In his mind, it was simply that the these relationships were more "impersonal" than his wife's.

Apart from coming for treatment because his wife wanted therapy for him, Benjamin was concerned about aging. He reported that his life lost its meaning momentarily and predictably when he was not busy professionally. This peculiar source of discomfort had plagued him since turning 50.

Testing

During his third month of treatment, Benjamin agreed to the Center's diagnostic assessment, which at that time consisted almost exclusively of personality tests and cognitive screening. Testing was delayed until the fourth month of treatment, when Benjamin could finally commit himself to continue with psychotherapy. The findings from that test battery were quite notable in the extent to which they conflicted with my clinical impressions and the degree to which this discrepancy persisted throughout treatment. In the end, this incongruity became our best clinical guide to Benjamin's personal reasons for remaining in while at the same time resisting treatment.

Judging from his professional accomplishments, Benjamin's intellect was flawless. On the 16 Personality Factors, a self-administered test that tends to emphasize personal strengths and scratches the psychological surface only, he emerged as independent, extroverted, and self-assured. In stark contrast, on the more deep-reaching self-report Minnesota Multiphasic Personality Inventory (MMPI) he appeared evasive and unable to admit personal flaws. Similarly, the Rorschach revealed difficulties with interpersonal closeness and an inclination to screen out complexity. Overall, according to the Rorschach, he was strikingly self-involved, supporting himself with defensive self-aggrandizement. His inflated sense of self was seen as disguising low self-esteem, bolstered characterlogically by constriction in his experience of emotions. The Rorschach ironically also revealed that he was very interested in and concerned about people, a picture most consistent with my clinical impression of him. Nonetheless, according to that test, he didn't understand people very well and was woefully lacking in intuition.

Pertinent Background

Benjamin's appraisal of his marriage and his relationship with his sons was notable in that, while according to his wife he had problems with intimacy, he originally claimed that his home life was nearly perfect. Still, Benjamin acknowledged that he always felt some inexplicable emotional distance from his wife and sons and was fundamentally at a loss about how to fully connect with them. Nonetheless, he viewed these relationships as successful, echoing his appraisal of most of the other important relationships in his life and reflecting his desire not to dig too deeply into imperfections.

Benjamin's parents were French-born Jews. They managed to find one another after their 3 years in Nazi work camps. He remembers both of them as being unrelentingly unemotional during his childhood. Emotions were never expressed in the home. His parents' philosophy was that "if you fall off a horse, you get back on it and don't stop to feel or think." While growing up, Benjamin's only "close" and constant relationship was with his 2-years-older sister. She is now an architect and lives in Texas.

Benjamin's father developed a successful business in the Midwest, providing his family with relative affluence. Benjamin attended a California college where he gained his "liberal" orientation, taking part in student protests during the 1960s. His father, who he admired and whose death he still grieves, died several years ago. Benjamin's mother now lives in Texas near his sister. He has trouble tolerating her erratic behavior and keeps his distance from her.

Presentation

Benjamin was affable, always acting as if everything in his life was perfectly okay. He was insistently, almost irritatingly, positive in describing his wife, sons, and friends, representing them all as nearly perfect. In addition to seeming unrealistic, this posture constantly made me worry about irritating him as I pushed for us to acknowledge and explore his troubles and reported deficits.

Our initial contract was for 1 year of treatment, later extended by Benjamin for 6 additional months. Benjamin originally agreed to the 1-year time limit as a strict condition for entering treatment. It was the maximum amount of time he was willing to devote to psychotherapy. Although extending treatment for 6 months at the end of the first year was presented by him as a concession to his wife, he acknowledged that, in addition to clarifying and addressing his problems with intimacy, therapy was mitigating his long-standing experience of emptiness when not fully occupied professionally.

Treatment

Sessions were organized around my pressing for Benjamin to become aware of his feelings through exercises noticing, feeling, and expressing emotions and my emphasizing the emotional complexity of his interactions with others, especially with me. I also strived to bring emotions into our relationship by informing him about how I was feeling in our interaction and simultaneously inquiring about his experience of being with me. To the degree that Benjamin allowed, we also regularly explored the origin of his lack of emotionality, particularly its basis in his parents' avoidance of all emotional expression during his childhood.

Benjamin would arrive each week having failed for the most part to do the exercises I suggested. When I noted his lack of compliance, his demeanor was generally vacant, as if the recommendations I made the previous week had never been given. He did acknowledge when he did not do them but generally let the matter drop at that point.

Frequently, Benjamin seemed on the verge of stopping treatment, leaving me feeling abandoned like his parents probably made him feel when during his childhood they failed to show emotion. In each of these sessions, I worked assiduously to bring Benjamin back, and by the end of the session he would usually be emotionally reengaged, leaving me feeling reasonably confident about our experience. I would comment about this shift, and he would concur that his experience had been similar. Nonetheless, for months his assent to be in and continue with therapy never felt very binding. I believe that it had a large element of acquiescence with my authority and his wife's dictum that he be in treatment with me. His lack of full involvement with treatment most likely was also based on Benjamin's not fully understanding the emotional depth we were striving for as reflected by his unrelenting claim that his life was already "perfect."

Benjamin's disconnection from treatment shifted dramatically after the feedback session following psychological testing, however. The feedback session became a nodal point heralding a dramatic shift in the therapy.

Both Dr. Engelman and I were present during this session.

Dr. Engelman began the session by summarizing the results of the testing in a straightforward manner. Benjamin responded with contempt saying that the results were "duh, no surprise at all." His hostility grew by the moment.

Taken aback, Dr. Engelman thoughtfully asked Benjamin how he thought that response made her feel. She then pressed the question, making Benjamin squirm since he suddenly became aware he might be offending her.

Rather than let Benjamin retract his response, I took control then and firmly but with feeling underscored the importance of Dr. Engelman's question. Apparently surprised at my passionate support of her, Benjamin slowly began to reflect but this time with growing animation. He was "shocked" at discovering that Dr. Engelman had "any feelings at all." In contrast to his usual emotional blandness, he became curious. What were the emotions she was talking about? Why hadn't he seen them? Where were his emotions? What part did he play in bringing out these seemingly unpleasant feelings in her?

From about that point, Benjamin began, for the first time, to show genuine interest in the test findings, especially those highlighting his difficulties understanding other people, their needs, and their emotions. He talked about his problems expressing and even feeling emotions, particularly in his relationships with his wife and children. He then requested two more sessions with Dr. Engelman and myself together. It was from that point, 6 months before the time-limited psychotherapy was to end, that he decided to work with me for an additional 6 months and soon thereafter to submit to retesting.

Limited Retesting 8 Months Later, Prior to Termination

After about 15 months of treatment, Benjamin requested retesting, this time in preparation for his likely termination. In addition to self-assessment questionnaires, he was given the MMPI and the Rorschach. The changes were striking. Presumably as a result of the therapy, Benjamin had become distinctly more introspective as well as better able to acknowledge his limitations and needs.

Termination

After vacation during the second summer of treatment, Benjamin came back saying that since we had worked together for the agreed-on year and a half, he had decided we should stop our work within a few sessions and that he would return to treatment if he found he needed it. It seemed judicious not to push my luck, and, as Benjamin requested, we stopped after three more sessions. At that point, he said that he was comfortable about what our psychotherapy had accomplished and that it would be better for him to be on his own, at least for a while.

Follow-Up

According to plan, I called Benjamin a few months after termination. We had a half hour conversation. He claimed that everything was fine, but in a way his statements sounded more like an evasion than a heartfelt report.

A year later, at his request, we met for a more extensive follow-up. At his suggestion, we met at a local coffeehouse. At that meeting, he was friendly and upbeat and said repeatedly that he appreciated our work together. This time, he seemed to mean it. He reported that his marriage, work, and relationships with his sons were distinctly improved as a result of the treatment. In contrast with our first follow-up conversation, he provided detail for these claims. He also said that because of continued discomfort about aging, he intended to return to psychotherapy, at least for a limited time.

Why Choose This as a Typical Case?

Why select this example as a typical "Center treatment"? The answer is that it is undistinguished. It incorporates elements found in most of our psychotherapies: assessment including appraisal of the patient's personal potential and failure to optimize that potential, personal struggle, ambivalence about commitment to treatment, and at least one nodal point during treatment marking the transition to a more productive therapy. The details of our assessment procedures and the treatments that follow can be found in chapters 5 and 6. Part of what makes this and other Center treatments distinctive is the use of psychological and neuropsychological assessment for ongoing guidance at the inception and then throughout the treatment and follow-up period. The involvement of a psychologist-assessor is itself a unique contribution to the assessment and treatment process. Adding to the richness of the therapy, the psychologist-assessor becomes an essential part of the psychotherapy team, repeatedly contributing his or her clinical observations as well as psychological and neuropsychological assessment findings to the therapy's guidance.

The Beginning or the End?

We are close to the end of this book. Yet, of course, our quest to understand how human beings can help one another change and how to maximize this change is never ending.

True, our next major project is to take the formal data that our diagnostics and monitoring yield and from these data derive effect sizes that we can compare to effect sizes from other studies. However, our outcome data will never fully qualify as well-constructed, adequately controlled research. Both to our benefit and to our detriment, in this project we are dealing with real-life people with actual problems, not research subjects who have been recruited for a study. It is often necessary for the guiding principles of a treatment to be adjusted over time. The data we used, while incorporating test results, were collaboratively processed between three people: the patient, therapist, and psychologist-assessor. More than anything, we want our work to count in the "real world," and we are aware that if we control treatment parameters too tightly, we run the risk losing the guts of the patient's dilemma and in effect losing track of the patient him- or herself (Norcross et al., 2006; Roth & Fonagy, 2005; Westen et al., 2004).

So, this is exactly where we believe we should be in this project—near the end yet repeatedly losing sight of it. If the end requires knowing what makes a psychotherapy effective, then I'm afraid we are left to contend with each case separately given the fact of its infinite and ever-shifting complexity.

In the next chapter, I summarize the position we have developed about psychotherapy and therapist accountability in chapters 1 through 8. Our stance is continually translated into the procedures and practices we use at the Center. As we learn, we change, so what you read here is already a bit outdated.

CHAPTER NINE

A New Paradigm for Psychotherapists?

What then have we come up with? Are we at the Center for Collaborative Psychology and Psychiatry proposing a truly different model for practice, in effect, a new paradigm? If we claim better accountability based on our diagnostic and monitoring procedures as well as the standard for practice that these hold for psychotherapy, on what grounds do we make this claim? Are the treatments we advocate readily accessible to office-based clinicians, and are they genuinely affordable?

Attempting to answer this question reminds me of my surprise when I recently picked up a book written in 1891 by Thomas Hardy. It contained a few irreverent expressions that I was sure that my generation had invented in the 1960s. Hardy's message is moderate and conventional but may have done its small part to contribute to later social change. The watershed of that change may have been in the 1960s. The 1960s was a time of earthshaking and apparently irreversible social and technological change. In addition to a technological revolution, there were radical shifts in thinking on almost every social front: profanity, music, marriage, sex, drugs, and child care, to name a few. Changes in how to think and behave as radical as these are uncommon in human experience. New adornment for already established cognitive paradigms is not (Kuhn, 1962).

In this book, I advocate what I believe is a new way of thinking about therapeutic procedure. It is not that all or even most of the components are new in themselves. Optimizing the reliability of clinical findings and therapist accountability are not novel ideas. It is the way the ingredients are chosen, thought about, and put together to achieve a result that may be. In our case, we emphasize therapist accountability for treatment progress, the regular use of psychological or neuropsychological testing, a vigorous collaborative dialogue between therapist and patient, heightened results through the kind of joining between therapist and patient that I call therapeutic conjunction (Frankel, 2007), and the inclusion of a psychologist-assessor as an integral member of the therapy team. The therapist in our model is not by any means a dispassionate observer, nor is he or she mainly a technician. He or she is most certainly both of these but also every bit a participant in the psychotherapeutic drama. He or she orchestrates treatment planning, takes responsibility for treatment effectiveness, contaminates the treatment with his or her emotions and prejudices, uses subjective data from the treatment to improve it, and, through his or energy and belief in the patient as well as psychological expertise, provides fuel for insight and change. The challenge has been to find ways the therapist can do and be in all these roles and bring each into play as needed.

So what have we really come up with? My guess is that by incorporating psychological and neuropsychological assessment in our initial and ongoing work, we have joined the quantitative virtues of the medical model and the subjective and interpersonal characteristics of the psychosocial. The product relies on and evolves according to a number of feedback mechanisms ranging from test data to personal judgment communicated between therapist and patient with and without words.

My objective in chapters 1 and 3 was to consider which nonspecific and specific factors optimize therapeutic work. My goal was to move us to think clearly about what measures are effective in psychosocial treatments. I wanted to undercut our tendency to make unsubstantiated claims about how much we accomplish as psychotherapists while at the same time, paradoxically, encouraging us as clinicians to recognize the potential power of our work.

In chapters 2, 4, 5, and 6, I elaborated methods of diagnosis and treatment monitoring we have developed and used at the Center. I applied those methods across the age spectrum from childhood through maturity, describing in chapter 7 the delivery of these services through the Center. The contribution I hope to make is in framing a method of diagnosis and treatment monitoring that psychotherapists can and will use: one that is office friendly and, over time, economically advantageous for the patient and family.

By using the phrase "economically advantageous," I do not mean to imply that testing is or should be cheap. The assessor needs to charge for his or her time and expenses, as does the therapist. True, in our assessment and monitoring procedures, we endeavor to restrict the number of tests we use and to remain cognizant of the costs of each. The real cost savings, however, comes from the guidance that the testing and second opinions from the psychologist-assessor repeatedly provide. Open-ended psychotherapy can be abysmally wasteful in both time and money. In some ways, its use is like trying to shoot with buckshot rather than with bullets from a gun with a sophisticated sighting device. Our claim is that with the assessment and monitoring techniques we recommend, a therapy is assured of being significantly more focused and productive. Of course, we need to substantiate these claims with more than just anecdotal examples, and that's just what these three projects are about.

What We Don't Know

There is a kind of illogic in the idea that we should be satisfied with the explanation that general, interpersonal factors do the lion's share of the work in psychotherapy. No doubt, they are powerful. Freud (1895) recognized that the laying on of hands could be remarkably healing for hysterical patients. But emotional problems often have their unique characteristics, each presumably best treated with specific techniques. When Damien, from chapter 8, was spinning out of control, the emotion was clearly rage that could quickly escalate, not some other emotion. He needed medication that would help him moderate his anger and behavioral techniques as well. Gary will tell you that the reason dialectical behavioral therapy was so helpful to him was that he needed to relearn certain behavior patterns. Reconfiguring his emotions, recognizing how anger erupted from experiences of betrayal, was helpful in a way that open-ended psychotherapy had not been. Being attuned and empathic would simply have not been enough in either case.

At the Center, we are alert to both sets of considerations: the contextual and the specific. Through collaborative feedback, we work with the patient to identify and make the adjustments needed for therapeutic accuracy. In effect, there are two pilots flying the aircraft, therapist and patient, each ready to hand the controls to the other. Periodic testing assures us that we have considered all the pertinent variables and helps us make major readjustments in our flight plan. The personalized contribution of subjectivity as well as distorted expectations based in transference and countertransference or errors in judgment are especially identified by testing and monitored by the third-person presence of the psychologist-assessor, who at times is our third pilot.

Imagine trying to fly a plane using three pilots. Yet, because our work is so heavily judgment based, we actually do best with these checks and balances in place. However, to avoid the most serious pitfall of this system, in the end we virtually always defer to the true flight leader: the patient. Ultimately, only he or she can determine fully where we are going and why. Any medical doctor will tell you that over time, a master practitioner generally becomes more realistic in acknowledging the limitations of diagnostic and prognostic precision in what he or she knows and does. Sorry, he or she would say, but a truly rigorous practitioner would never promise a magic bullet. Nor would this doctor be likely to denigrate out of hand alternative treatments, such as aspects of herbal remedies or acupuncture, that haven't yet been subjected to the scrutiny of randomized controlled trials. He or she would simply add that the efficacy of these treatments remains to be demonstrated. After all, is my hyperrealistic neighbor Roberta out of her mind when she claims that her headaches were for the first time controlled by the Ayurvedic principles of Indian medicine and when she insists that the effect is real, not due to a placebo factor?

While we as psychotherapists rarely have clinically pertinent medical tests and radiological imaging to orient us, we do have psychological and neuropsychological testing. Additionally, with the subjective report that we are privileged to get as we speak with the patient, we may gain a pretty good idea about how he or she is thinking, what other factors are at play in his or her life, what supports are available to him or her, and whether he or she is being fully compliant with and interested in the treatment. We also are likely to have a good read on the patient's ability to prevail under duress. Blood levels aren't everything, after all. In general medicine, doctors frequently do not have the time or even interest to tune into either the real or the subjective aspects of a patient's life (Charon, 2006; Frankel, Quill, & McDaniel, 2003).

In chapters 1 through 4, we considered the knotty issue of whether psychotherapy as a psychosocial intervention works and, if so, how well. Strikingly, the data on this subject pretty much argue for the value of psychotherapy and the place of contextual factors in its effectiveness. While this is a politically loaded issue and appears to be the basis of a bitter territorial dispute between at least some psychologists who hold tenaciously to the contextual model and those psychiatrists who are particularly fixed on their identity as physicians, the research, the statistical analyses, and the meta-analyses (Smith, Glass, & Miller, 1980; Wampold, 2001) speak for themselves. No matter how much we are in love with empirically supported treatments (ESTs) given their origins in double-blind controlled studies, the long-term outcome from most EST protocols are not substantiated, just preferred by the more scientific among us (Fonagy, Target, Cottrell, Phillips, & Kurtz, 2002; Jacobson & Christensen, 1996a, 1996b; Norcross, Beutler, &

Levant, 2006; Roth & Fonagy, 2005; Westen, Novotny, & Thompson-Brenner, 2004).

At its heart, psychotherapy is with people, not automatons. People are social animals. Ordinarily, they need to feel acknowledged and understood to be motivated to make personal changes. The old psychoanalytic notion of "resistance" to meaningful involvement in treatment and, implicitly therefore, to change is actually alive and well in ways. People are complex and generally have multiple agendas moving them, many of which they are unaware. These unconscious or dissociated schemas (Bromberg, 1994, 1998), take your choice which concept you prefer, are indeed a major part of the purview of depth psychotherapy. And yet, as I assert in chapter 3, EST is truly alive and well. In fact, EST provides a welcome corrective to our traditional intuition-guided practices and their inadequate attention to defining and rigorously following therapeutic progress.

Clearly, at this point we need more information on what specific behavioral and biological interventions work and why. These are the techniques used over and above the interpersonal-contextual influences required for any psychotherapy to be effective. Included in this inquiry must be a longitudinal look at what to expect from each of these treatments, longitudinal since we know that treatment effects, especially if unreinforced, tend to fade over time and merge with those of other interventions (Mueller et al., 1999; Westen et al., 2004). The gratuitous claims by drug company–supported investigations that particular medications are effective, for example, may come from poorly designed, inadequately controlled, relatively short-term studies. The reader is referred to Stein, Lerer, and Stahl's (2005) review of evidence-based psychopharmacology to see what has actually been demonstrated about the efficacy of each class of drugs. Remarkably, the research currently available remains inconclusive in almost every psychopharmacological category. In most cases, it is unclear which drugs are superior, if and what combination of pharmacotherapy and psychotherapy is likely to be optimal, how long treatments should last, and what is the most desirable maintenance regime. A few exceptions to this generalization include the established benefit of cognitive-behavioral treatments for phobias, the place of traditional and newer neuroleptics in the treatment of schizophrenia and bipolar manic episodes, the anxiolytic and antidepressant effects of serotonin- and norepinephrine-enhancing antidepressants, and the effectiveness of stimulants for attentional disorders. Finally, there is evidence, albeit more tentative, for the value of other mood-stabilizing drugs and antipsychotics in the treatment and prophylaxis for bipolar disorder, especially mania. Of the mood stabilizers, lithium is the most well researched and clinically established pharmacological treatment for bipolar disorder, especially mania. Also, while in many clinical situations the superiority of pharmacotherapy over psychosocial interventions is not clearly established, it often seems wise to use both when they are available (Pinquart, Duberstein, & Lyness, 2006; Plunkin, 2006; Roth & Fonagy, 2005).

Yet it would be absurd to understate the place of medication in the treatment of psychiatric entities such as schizophrenia, depression, attention deficit disorder, and bipolar illness. True, their use in psychiatric disturbance altogether and in sleep regulation may be less precisely characterized at this point than is ideal. All behavior has a biological, biochemical, and genetic basis. Those realities make it is hard to imagine that biological treatments should be a secondary consideration, dwarfed by Wampold's (2001) contextual considerations when accounting for therapeutic success. I believe this point holds in spite of the fact that no psychopharmacologist I know of would claim that at this point we can pinpoint most biological interventions to fit a specific patient and his or her disorder. In the end, each patient is at least a little bit different biochemically and genetically. Our knowledge in this area is simply not yet specific enough to predict which patient requires exactly which drugs and in what quantities. In fact, the same statement can be made about most areas of medicine as well, where precise diagnosis and treatment are often confounded by comorbid medical and even psychiatric conditions or simply by imprecision in the way treatment is formulated and paced.

The Person Factor

Whatever our convictions, the bottom line is that we are practicing in the world as clinicians and know that, in treatment, hands on truly makes a difference. This generalization applies in physical medicine no less than in psychotherapy. As psychotherapists, we see remarkable transformations in people's moods and habits that are not directly attributable to biological factors.

For one thing, whatever else we do, beyond addressing the patient's main complaints, we usually help our patients by anticipating what and how much they can accomplish. These expectations are formulated using history, psychological and neuropsychological assessment data, collaborative input from the patient, and our own intuition and experience. They are communicated between the patient and therapist both verbally and nonverbally. This communication as much explains change in most psychotherapies as do other therapeutic interventions, specific or contextual. The therapist develops an educated impression of the patient's wishes and potential, a picture of who the patient is, how much he or she can heal him- or herself, and what of his or her personal goals he or she can achieve. Formulating these expectations requires a highly refined appraisal, arrived at collaboratively between therapist and patient, rendered as much to intuition as consciousness and incorporated into the way the therapist behaves. The result is a tribute to the beneficial effect people can have on one another. The patient gets a green light, and seemingly out of thin air there is a burst of renewed and new personal development (Frankel, 2007). Call it what you want, but this sudden jolt forward often feels like magic.

After all, going back to chapter 1, just what did Dr. Crane do in Dori's treatment to release her back into real life? For the record, I hear that she is now happier and more productive than ever before in her life. Recall the extent to which her depression had crippled her. Add to that report the fact that her two seasoned previous psychotherapists were unable to help her. Finally, consider that Dr. Crane treated Dori with so much respect, apparently expecting that with a bit of help Dori would find her own way. From what I gather, her previous therapists were themselves alarmed by the magnitude of Dori's anxiety and treated her like a psychological cripple.

At this point, I want to restate our professional dilemma. One place I believe many of us as psychotherapists tend to get stuck is in our need to feel effective. Underpinning this requirement is often the conviction that we as individuals are unique in our ability to understand and help people, an assumption that may in fact have brought us into the helping professions in the first place. One of the least comfortable experiences for us as psychotherapists is when we are forced to face our uncertainty about how and why we select a particular treatment strategy, how well it will work, or even if it will work at all. Medical doctors and psychiatrists who rely primarily on biological or combined biological and behavioral methods can, for the most part, sidestep this uncertainty. However, hidden in this sometimes slippery stance is often reliance on data that may not be reliable and that, for example, may be tainted by unsubstantiated claims (Healy, 2005; Stein et al., 2005). Commonly, this stance is predicated on a belief that numbers are a safer haven than the usual more complex subjectivity-infused information we have about the human being who is our patient.

The Gospel Truth and What to Do About It

Added to the more concrete factors influencing claims about psychotherapy efficacy is psychological gospel. Regardless of the tradition in which we were trained, whether biological, Jungian, behavioral, Freudian,

Kleinian, Fairbairnian, or even an eclectic mixture of several of these, we have generally been told that we have received some version of the truth. Some form of genuflecting is often part of the prescribed practice, the belief that if you have the truth, you need to repeatedly cleanse yourself of contaminating ideas. Some of you, I imagine, will be starting to feel irritated at me at this point and will be thinking something like, "Come off it Frankel, I'm above that." And with some luck and a lot of wisdom, you indeed may be. But institutional pull is insidious and unbelievably powerful. When the hard questions about one's therapeutic convictions are asked, a painful reckoning often descends, as it did with me just after I completed my psychoanalytic training. At that point, I had to ask whether I really believed that psychoanalysis as a treatment was more effective than therapies carried out less frequently or whether treatment on the couch worked better than treatment face-to-face. How did my psychoanalytic teachers and supervisors arrive at their convictions about the superiority of psychoanalysis? Since most of what they learned themselves was based on assertions passed on by teachers, what made those educators so willing to accept them as established truths?

The fate of Freud's theories and original practices is a conventional example of observations that became dogma. While eloquently and even modestly presented by him in his writing, these theories were, after all, derived retrospectively from clinical data. While he was flexible enough to revise his formulations over the course of his professional lifetime, he did progressively demand strict adherence from his group of supporters and was progressively unforgiving in his insistence on their ideological compliance (Fromm, 1970; Jung, 1975). The "wrong" belief system could land you outside the swinging door. Incidentally, as so often happens, his disciples became much more rigid than Freud. In Freud's hands, psychoanalysis was often completed in months, and there was room for semiformal encounters with the patient, several of whom accompanied Freud while he was on summer retreat. Somehow the standard for a successful analysis and especially a training analysis were soon expanded to four or even five sessions a week, lasting for an undefined period of years. Criteria for a successful analysis were vague and related to an elusive development in the treatment called a transference neurosis.

A personal vignette may help elaborate my point. While remaining politically unaligned, I had one of these swinging-door experiences at the traditional psychoanalytic institute where I was trained. After I had been teaching a popular seminar at the institute for 6 years, one of the more conservative training analysts caught on to my relational bias. At the end of that academic year, I received a formal but polite letter saying that, according to (more often than not violated) institute rules, courses were not to be taught for more than 6 years (thank you very much, Dr. F.). Had that been the usual fate of other instructor-colleagues, I would have believed the offered explanation. Happily, I was able to get this decision reversed. Finding out what really happened in creating this decision required sleuth work. Sadly, it turned out that the move to eliminate my rather avant-garde seminar on human development from the syllabus had been due mainly to the work of a few old "friends." They were fervently attempting to consolidate their traditional psychoanalytic hold on the Institute as new ideas were beginning to pour in (Kuhn, 1962). Oddly, as early as the next year, I was asked to run for the presidency of the institute. Apparently, that choice was in part based on my reputation for keeping free of institute politics.

Ironically, as necessity has dictated and as psychoanalysis has become less popular, the rules of psychoanalytic training have been loosened at most psychoanalytic institutes. It is okay to convert a patient from psychotherapy to psychoanalysis now, to see patients fewer times a week than in the past, and to judiciously dispense with the couch. The psychoanalytic literature is replete with references to the "real relationship," a change that must have Franz Alexander reveling in his grave. During his lifetime, Alexander was made into a pariah by mainstream psychoanalysts for advocating such an idea. In those days, references to the real relationship were guarded (Alexander & French, 1946; Greenacre, 1971; Greenson, 1971), and the notion that part of what psychoanalysis provided was a "corrective emotional experience" was for the most part unacceptable.

So, if gospel is so context dependent, in what can a therapist believe? What information, what assessments, provide the kind of definitive data that any principled professional needs to have to be sure that he is providing not just the right but also the optimal psychotherapy?

One quick answer, of course, is to use the procedures we have developed at the Center. The complexity of each intervention, its ever-changing nature, and the unique requirements of each patient are precisely the reasons for the way we have designed the Center's procedure. It needed to be flexible, sorting between a plethora of diagnostic possibilities, and available to follow the patient throughout the treatment to determine if the therapy is succeeding and what modifications might be required.

What We Still Need to Know

The therapist's ideology aside, if the limits of our psychiatric and medical assessments are built into what we see and do as practitioners, what information about the nature and progress of a therapy can we rely on, and to what degree? How far can our observations and clinical judgments carry us? It is interesting that as I end this book, much of what I am left with are questions. Honestly, I did not anticipate—yet I am intrigued by—this outcome.

In chapter 3, I made the literature-supported (Kubiszyn et al., 2000; Meyer, 2003; Meyer et al., 2001) assertion that assessment in psychiatry and psychology may not be any less accurate than its equivalent in physical medicine, especially when it is interpreted and used by an experienced practitioner. Of course, this generalization is counterintuitive. So we are left with the question of whether it is true, to what extent, and for which kinds of psychological and psychiatric assessments.

There are several literature reviews and metapsychological studies (Lambert, 2004; Norcross et al., 2006; Smith, Glass, & Miller, 1980; Wampold, 2001) that conclude that treatment with psychotherapy has unequivocally been shown to be of significant clinical benefit. Here too, there may be influences that could distort the authors' positions. For example, to what extent is psychotherapy advocacy politically biased? What are the dissenting arguments against this psychotherapy-friendly stance as reflected in the common psychiatric assertion that biological considerations should be given precedence over interpersonal ones? Can so many physicians and others who support ESTs be so misguided that they cling for dear life to a belief system that is false?

Even if one takes the view that psychotherapy is clearly effective, the literature (Lambert, 2004; Westen et al., 2004) is still impressively unsettled in so many areas. To cite a few, what difference do the following make? (a) the therapist's experience and training (Christensen & Jacobson, 1996b; Miller & Binder, 2002; Sandell et al., 2006; Stein & Lambert, 1995), (b) the duration and frequency of sessions both for biological and psychosocial treatments (Barkham et al., 1996a, 1996b; Crits-Cristoph, 1992), and (c) the theoretical orientation of the treating person and the techniques selected by him or her (Barrett & Berman, 2001; Beutler & Harwood, 2000; Frank & Frank, 1991; Howard et al., 1996; Malik, Alimohamed, Holoway, & Beutler, 2000; Roussos, Lisson, & De Duarte, 2007). Also, what is there to say about the potential power of friendship and of inspiration (Gould & Clum, 1993)? Can they substitute for or even equal the benefits of psychotherapy?

As an example of the lack of clarity in these areas, Westen et al. (2004) as well as Norcross et al. (2006) cite metapsychological data holding that the impact of training on outcome is minimal, except in situations requiring unique technical skills from the psychotherapist. In contrast to these reviews, some individual studies (Bein et al., 2000; Hilsenroth, 2007) do suggest that the quality of a therapist's training is related to improved therapy results, but these are relatively small studies, each specific to the kinds of training and psychotherapy being evaluated, and cannot be considered conclusive.

What to believe? Personally, it is hard for me to imagine that the benefits of training are so limited. Common sense does not support that view. True, research data suggest that that may be the case. However, relatively unaccounted for in the literature reviews I have read is the depth of a therapist's training and the impact of his or her clinical experience on therapy outcome, variables likely to be difficult or even impossible to quantify. After all, if we are focusing on equivalences between medical and psychosocial practice, can you imagine, after months of progressive chest pain, going to a heart specialist who has not done a fellowship at a credible training center and who does not have years of frontline experience?

Also, what kinds of assessment tools are most useful and for what kinds of psychological and psychiatric conditions? At what points in treatment are these assessments likely to be most revealing? This topic is addressed but not with clinical specificity in the Meyer et al. (2001) article and again by Meyer (2003). To what extent can psychological test findings be relied on over time, and how quickly and basically can results from each type of assessment shift as the patient's frame of mind and physical status change? Cole, Martin, Powers, and Truglio (1996), Meyer et al. (2001), and Millon (1996) are among the many psychologists who advocate multimethod assessment, with each of two or more parallel assessments acting as a check on the others. Accepting that multimethod assessment, including the input of a psychologist-assessor within the three-person field and the self-assessment provided by the therapist and patient collaboration, is a helpful truing mechanism for psychotherapy, what other truing mechanisms are there?

What are the effects of cultural and temperamental factors on the validity of clinical judgment and assessment? (For a thoughtful review related to this subject, see Weinberger & Westen, 2004.) Can these factors be missed by assessment instruments? In particular, which tests are likely to fail in these areas?

How accurately can subtle, intangible influences bolstering the patient's identity, personal strengths, and potential and basic attitudes such as trust be identified either through clinical judgment or by using formal psychological and neuropsychological testing? Note that so much of what a therapist does—and of what I am calling therapeutic and assessment acrobatics and magic—involves facilitating the enhancement and consolidation of these factors (Frankel, 1995, 2000, 2007). Intangible means undetected, not consciously apparent to the patient and especially the therapist. These developments in treatment are usually hard to identify and characterize. They often are not deliberately orchestrated. However, my impression is that they are frequently intuitively appreciated, planned, and even contrived by the therapist and patient.

Further, the dialogue between therapist and patient, the nuts and bolts of the "magic" to which I refer, is not amorphous in nature, as the terms *intuitive* and *clinical judgment* may suggest. It is consists of a complex mix of split-second emotional responsiveness and cognitive agility. Psychosocial interventions, their sometimes magical-seeming outcomes, require therapist and patient to take personal and interpersonal risks in their judgment and actions. In my opinion, it would be absurd to imagine that the accuracy of the therapist's judgment in this process is not enhanced by his or her training and clinical as well as life experience.

Returning to Dori from chapter 1, clearly Dr. Crane's ability to understand her reflected remarkably astute clinical judgment. She got it right where Dori's other therapists had failed. All three therapists were well trained, and all believed they were the right person to help Dori. However, the first two, Thea and Wanda, apparently lacked both the humility and the judgment to understand just what Dori needed. The evidence for this assertion is straightforward. With both of the early therapists, Dori failed to progress and even frankly deteriorated; with Dr. Crane, she soared.

Or, for that matter, how did Dr. Engelman decide when to make her groundbreaking observation of Benjamin's interpersonal obtuseness as reflected in his indifference to her sensibilities? How did she know that it would be just that observation, said at just that moment, that he would hear? Or how did I decide to challenge Gary's claim that his bipolarity was incurable? His very identity was based on his belief that he had a disabling, in fact incurable, psychiatric disorder. In both instances, the therapist had to take a risk that, according to the patient's treatment history, could have brought on a storm of criticism and anger, causing the therapy to crash into smithereens.

So what is clinical judgment (Baker, 2001; Haynes, Devereaux, & Guyatt, 2002; Parry, Cape, & Pilling, 2003, Weinberger & Westen, 2004)? How is it kept on target? To what extent are medical and/or psychological tests able to assist with the significantly intuitive process of clinical judgment, and at which points in a diagnostic procedure and treatment? What difference do training, clinical and life experience, intelligence, and common sense make for the accuracy of clinical judgment? How much distortion is introduced by each player: therapist and patient? How does the role of clinical judgment in psychosocial treatment, in the absence of psychological test data, compare to that in general medicine, where blood tests and scans are almost always available?

Where We Are Left

It seems most fitting to end this book with a series of questions. It is not simply that much research remains to be done. Taking that position would suggest that most of these questions have an answer. True, somewhere there may be reasonably clear answers to the issue of what makes a psychotherapy effective at any single point. But even by the next day, there are likely to be new, influential developments in that patient's life, biochemical shifts, and mood changes. Then there is the therapist's spontaneous reactions to the patient. Whether or not it is comfortable for us to accept, we like or love some patients and feel repulsed by others. To make matters more complicated, each patient brings an entirely new set of objective and subjective parameters to the therapy, even if his or her diagnosis is the same as that of others. Two patients who are ostensibly alike may have dissimilar backgrounds. They may have vastly different personal, professional, or financial resources and thus different reasons for being in treatment. They may have different tolerances for the requirements of psychotherapy, including the required self-reflection and collaboration with the therapist. And, most certainly, they may have different aspirations.

There are ways to search for answers, however. While likely to shift, even radically, during a therapy, these truing methods consist of collaboration between the therapist and patient and assessments that monitor diagnosis as well as regression and progress. At each point, they can be used to keep the therapist and patient on track in treatment and to bring themselves into alignment.

Sound exhausting? Or does it instead sound exciting, opening the possibilities for other ways to understand the patient?

Here, of course, is where creativity comes it. The most exciting outcome of our investigation of what makes psychotherapy work is actually that there are usually myriad alternative ways of therapist and patient acting, of creating novel and even distinctly better outcomes. But how novel is novel? As we do our work as psychotherapists, will we simply repeat old formulas or on occasion actually come up with new paradigms for seeing and acting?

The Future

Where to go from here? Is psychotherapy, whether interpersonal or behavioral, alive and promising, or is it dying and stale?

That question of the fate of psychotherapy may not be very different from how much personal help one individual can provide another. After all, where else could help come from if not another human being? Given our clinical experience and what we have read in the psychotherapy research literature, the answer of course is that psychotherapy used alone or in combination with other measures such as medication is quite alive as well as exciting, challenging, and remarkably promising. Recommending psychotherapy itself, apart from its other virtues, is its relative safety as compared with medications and other biologically based interventions, especially when psychotherapy is practiced with humility. It becomes dangerous or destructive only when the practitioner becomes punitive, too certain about the truth of his or her belief system, or intoxicated with authority.

We at the Center are constantly collating data from the testing of our patients. Phil Erdberg and I are working hard with such data to understand what actually happens in an effective psychotherapy, at which points and with whom. We want to pinpoint the creative moments and when and how the most important shifts occur. We are working to determine how to concentrate key therapeutic factors so that psychotherapy is optimally reliable and effective. We are particularly interested in understanding the powerful, often magical seeming spontaneous changes we often observe during psychotherapy (Frankel, 2007).

We are excited as we search for theoretical and clinical enlightenment. We hope you are as well.

Please do tune in again soon.

Bibliography

Addis, M. E. (1997). Evaluating the treatment manual as a means of disseminating empirically validated psychotherapies. *Clinical Psychology: Science and Practice, 4,* 1–11.

Addis, M. E. (2002). Methods for disseminating research products and increasing evidence-based practice: Promises, obstacles, and future directions. *Clinical Psychology: Science and Practice,* 9, 381–392.

Addis, M. E., Hatgis, C., Krasnow, A. D., Jacob, K., Bourne, L., & Mansfield, A. (2004). Effectiveness of cognitive-behavioral treatment for panic disorder versus treatment as usual in a managed care setting. *Journal of Consulting and Clinical Psychology, 72,* 625–635.

Addis, M. E., & Krasnow, A. D. (2002). A national survey of practicing psychologists' attitudes toward psychology treatment manuals. *Journal of Consulting and Clinical Psychology,* 68, 331–339.

Alberts, G., & Edelstein, B. (1990). Therapist training: A critical review of skill training studies. *Clinical Psychology Review, 10,* 497–511.

Alexander, F., & French, T. M. (1946). *Psychoanalytic therapy: Principles and application.* New York: Ronald Press.

American Psychological Association. (2002a). Criteria for evaluating treatment guidelines. *American Psychologist, 57,* 1052–1059.

American Psychological Association. (2002b). Criteria for practice guideline development and evaluation. *American Psychologist, 57,* 1048–1051.

American Psychological Association Task Force on the Promotion and Dissemination of Psychological Procedures. (1995). Training in a dissemination of empirically-validated psychological treatments: Report and recommendations. Criteria for practice guideline development and evaluation. *Clinical Psychologist,* 48, 3–23.

Aron, L. (1991). The patient's experience of the analyst's subjectivity. *Psychoanalytic Dialogues, 1*(1), 29–51.

Aron, L. (1992). Interpretation as expression of the analyst's subjectivity. *Psychoanalytic Dialogues, 2*(4), 475–508.

Aron, L. (1996). *A meeting of the minds: Mutuality in psychoanalysis*. Hillsdale, NJ: Analytic Press.

Auerhahn, N., & Peskin, H. (2003). Action knowledge, acknowledgement, and interpretive action in work with Holocaust survivors. *Psychoanalytic Quarterly, 72*, 445–456.

Bachrach, H., Galatzer-Levy, R., Skolnikoff, A., & Waldron, S. (1991). On the efficacy of psychoanalysis. *Journal of the American Psychoanalytic Association, 39*, 871–914.

Baker, R. (2001). Is it time to review the idea of compliance with guidelines? *British Journal of General Practice, 51*, 7.

Barber, J. P., Connolly, M. B., Crits-Christoph, P., Gladis, L., & Siqueland, L. (2000). Alliance predicts patients' outcome beyond in-treatment change in symptoms. *Journal of Consulting and Clinical Psychology*, 68, 1027–1032.

Barkham, M., Rees, A., Shapiro, D. A., Stiles, W. B., Agnew, R. M., Halstead, J., et al. (1996a). Outcomes of time-limited psychotherapy in applied settings: Replicating the second Sheffield psychotherapy project. *Journal of Consulting and Clinical Psychology*, 64, 1079–1085.

Barkham, M., Rees, A., Stiles, W. B., Shapiro, D. A., Hardy, G. E., & Reynolds, S. (1996b). Dose effect relations in time limited psychotherapy for depression. *Journal of Consulting and Clinical Psychology*, 64, 927–935.

Barlow, D. (1988). Treatment outcome evaluation methodology with anxiety disorder: Strengths, and statistical considerations. *Advances in Behavior Research and Therapy, 11*, 121–132.

Barlow, D., & Hayes, S. (1979). Alternating treatment design: One strategy for comparing the effects of two treatments in a single subject. *Journal of Applied Behavior Analysis, 12*, 199–210.

Barrett, M. S., & Berman, J. (2001). Is psychotherapy more effective when therapists disclose information about themselves? *Journal of Consulting and Clinical Psychology*, 69, 597–603.

Barrowclough, C., Kind, P., Colville, J., Russell, E., Burns, A., & Tarrier, N. (2001). A randomized trial of the effectiveness of cognitive-behavioral therapy and supportive counseling for anxiety symptoms in older adults. *Journal of Consulting and Clinical Psychology*, 69, 756–762.

Beach M. C., & Inui, T. S. (2006). Relationship-centered care: A constructive reframing. *Journal of General Internal Medicine, 21*, S3–S8.

Beck, A. T. (1976). *Cognitive therapy and emotional disorders*. New York: International Universities Press.

Bein, E., Anderson, T., Strupp, H. H., Henry, W., Schacht, T. E., Binder, J. L., et al. (2000). The effects of training in time-limited dynamic psychotherapy: Changes in therapeutic outcome. *Psychotherapy Research, 10*(2), 119–132.

Beutler, L. E., Engle, D., Mohr, D., Daldrup, R. J., Bergan, J., Meredith, K., et al. (1991). Predictors of differential response to cognitive, experiential, and self-directed psychotherapeutic procedures. *Journal of Consulting and Clinical Psychology,* 59, 333–340.

Beutler, L. E., & Harwood, T. M. (2000). *Prescriptive psychotherapy.* New York: Oxford University Press.

Block, J., & Block, J. (1973). *Ego development and the provenance of thought: A longitudinal study of ego and cognitive development in young children.* Berkeley: University of California Press.

Block, J., & Block, J. (1980). The role of ego-control and ego-resiliency in the organization of behavior. In W. A. Collins (eds), *Minnesota Symposium on Child Psychology: vol 13. Development of cognition, affect, and social relations* (pp. 39–101). Hillsdale, N.J.: Erlbaum.

Bohart, A. (2005). Evidence-based psychotherapy means evidence informed, not evidence-driven. *Journal of Contemporary Psychotherapy,* 35, 39–53.

Bromberg, P. (1994). "Speak! that I may see you": Some reflections on dissociation, reality and psychoanalytic listening. *Psychoanalytic Dialogues,* 4, 517–547.

Bromberg, P. (1996). *Standing in the spaces: Essays on clinical process, trauma, and dissociation.* Hillsdale, NJ: Analytic Press.

Bromberg, P. (1998). Standing in spaces: The multiplicity of self and the psychoanalytic relationship. *Contemporary Psychoanalysis, 32,* 509–536.

Campbell, J. M. (2004). Statistical comparisons of four effect sizes for single-subject designs. *Behavior Modification, 28,* 234–246.

Castonguay, L. G., Schut, A. J., Constantino, M. J., & Halperin, G. S. (1999). Assessing the role of treatment manuals: Have they become necessary but nonsufficient ingredients of change? *Clinical Psychology: Science and Practice,* 6, 449–455.

Chambless, D. L., & Hollon, S. D. (1998). Defining empirically supported therapies. *Journal of Consulting and Clinical Psychology,* 64, 497–504.

Chambless, D., & Hollon, S. D. (2002). Cognitive therapy and pharmacotherapy for depression: Singly or in combination. *Archives of General Psychiatry,* 49, 774–781.

Chambless, D. L., & Ollendick, T. H. (2001). Empirically supported psychological interventions: Controversies and evidence. *Annual Review of Psychology, 52,* 685–716.

Chambless, D. L., Sanderson, W., Shoham, V., Johnson, S., Pyne, J., & Pope, K. (1996). An update on empirically validated therapies. *The Clinical Psychologist,* 49, 5–18.

Chambless, D. L., Sanderson, W., Shoham, V., Johnson, S., Pyne, J., & Pope, K. (1998). Update on empirically validated therapies, II. *The Clinical Psychologist, 51,* 3–16.

Charon, R. (2006). *Families, systems and health: Vol. 23. Narrative medicine: Honoring the stories of illness.* New York: Oxford University Press.

Chused, J. (1991). The evocative power in enactments. *Journal of the American Psychoanalytic Association, 39*(3), 615–639.

Cole, D. A., Martin, J, Powers, B., & Truglio, R. (1996). Modeling casual relations between academic and social competence and depression: A multitrait-multimethod longitudinal study of children. *Journal of Abnormal Psychology, 105*, 258–270.

Crits-Cristoph, P. (1992). The efficacy of brief dynamic psychotherapy: A meta-analysis. *American Journal of Psychiatry, 149*, 151–158.

Crits-Cristoph, P., Wilson, G., & Hollon, S. (2005) Empirically supported psychotherapies: Comment on Westen, Novotny, and Thompson-Brennen (2004). *Psychological Bulletin, 131*, 412–417.

Davidson, K. W., Goldstein, M., Kaplan, R. M., Kaufmann, P. G., Knatterud, G. L., Orleans, C. T., et al. (2003). Evidence-based behavioral medicine. What is it, and how do we achieve it? *Annual of Behavioral Medicine*, 26, 161–171.

Degury, F. (2003). A biopsychosocial perspective on mental disorders: Depression in the primary care setting. In Frankel, R., Quill, T., & McDaniel, S. (Eds.), *The biopsychosocial approach: Past, present, and future* (pp. 82–90). Rochester, NY: University of Rochester Press.

Duffy, F., & Gordon, G. (2004). Assessment of competency in interpersonal and communication skills: Kalamazoo II. *Academic Medicine, 79*(6), 495–507.

Elkin, I., Shea, M., Watkins, H., Imber, S., Sotsky, S., Collins, J., et al. (1989). National Institute of Mental Health Treatment of Depression Collaborative Research Program: General effectiveness of treatments. *Archives of General Psychiatry*, 46, 971–982.

Engelman, D., & Frankel, S. (2002). The three person field: Collaborative consultation to psychotherapy. *The Humanistic Psychologist*, 30, 49–62.

Epstein, R. (1995). Communication between primary care physicians and consultants. *Archives of Family Medicine, 37*, 377–388.

Erikson, E. (1968). *Identity: Youth and crisis.* New York: Norton.

Finn, S. (2007). *In our clients' shoes: Theory and techniques of therapeutic assessment.* Mahwah, NJ: Lawrence Erlbaum Associates.

Finn, S., & Fischer, C. (1997, August 18). *Therapeutic psychological assessment: Illustration and analysis of philosophical assumptions.* Presented at the annual meeting of the American Psychological Association, Chicago, IL.

Fischer, C. (1994). *Individualizing psychological assessment.* Mahwah, NJ: Lawrence Erlbaum Associates. (Original work published 1985)

Fischer, C. (2000). Collaborative individualized assessment. *Journal of Personality Assessment, 74*, 2–14.

Fisher, J., & O'Donohue, W. (Eds.). (2006). *A practitioner's guide to evidence-based psychotherapy.* New York: Springer.

Flavell, J. (1963). *The developmental psychology of Jean Piaget*. New York: Van Nostrand Reinhold.

Fonagy, P., Target, M., Cottrell, D., Phillips, J., & Kurtz, Z. (2002). *What works for whom: A critical review of treatments for children and adolescents*. New York: Guilford Press.

Frank, J. D., & Frank, J. B. (1991). *Persuasion and healing* (3rd ed.). Baltimore: Johns Hopkins University Press.

Frankel, R., & Gerrity, M. (2007). Re-forming relationships in health care. *Journal of General Internal Medicine, 21*(Suppl. 1), S1–S47.

Frankel, R., & Inui, T. (2006). Reforming relationships in health care. *Journal of General Internal Medicine, 21*, S1–S2.

Frankel, R., Quill, T., & McDaniel, S. (2003). *The biopsychosocial approach: Past, present, and future*. Rochester, NY: University of Rochester Press.

Frankel, S. (1995). *Intricate engagements: The collaborative basis of therapeutic change*. Northvale, NJ: Jason Aronson.

Frankel, S. (2000). *Hidden faults: Recognizing and resolving therapeutic disjunctions*. Madison, CT: International Universities Press.

Frankel, S. (2006). The clinical use of therapeutic disjunctions. *Psychoanalytic Psychotherapy, 23*, 56–71.

Frankel, S. (2007). *Making psychotherapy work: Collaborating successfully with your patient*. Madison, CT: International Universities Press.

Freud, S. (1895). The psychotherapy of hysteria. In S. Freud & J. Breuer, *Studies in hysteria* (pp. 299–352.). New York: Avon.

Fromm, E. (1970). *The crisis of psychoanalysis: Essays on Freud, Marx, and social psychology*. Greenwich, CT: Fawcett.

Garfinkel, H. (1967). *Studies in ethnomethodology*. Englewood Cliffs, NJ: Prentice Hall.

Gerth, H., & Mills, C. (1946). *From Max Weber: Essays in sociology*. New York: Oxford University Press.

Ghaemi, S. (2002). *Polypharmacy in psychiatry*. New York: Marcel Dekker.

Ghaemi S., & Hsu, D. (2005). Evidence-based pharmacology of bipolar disorder. In D. Stein, B. Lerer, & S. Stahl (Eds.), *Evidence-based psychopharmacology* (pp. 22–25). Cambridge: Cambridge University Press.

Goebel-Fabbri, A. E., Fikkan, J., & Franko, D. L. (2003). Beyond the manual: The flexible use of cognitive behavioral therapy. *Cognitive and Behavioral Practice, 10*, 41–50.

Gould, R. A., & Clum, G. A. (1993). A meta-analysis of self-help treatment approaches. *Clinical Psychology Review, 13*, 169–186.

Greenacre, P. (1971). *Emotional growth* (Vol. 2). New York: International Universities Press.

Greenfield, S., & Kaplan, S. (1985). Expanding patient involvement in care: Effects on patient outcomes. *Annals of Internal Medicine, 102*(4), 520–528.

Greenson, R. (1978). The "real" relationship between the patient and the psychoanalyst. In *Explorations in psychoanalysis* (pp. 115–158). New York: International Universities Press.

Grossman, L. (1996). The analyst's influence. *Psychoanalytic Quarterly*, *65*, 681–692.

Grotstein, J. (1981). *Splitting and projective identification*. New York: Jason Aronson.

Hamilton, C. (2000) Continuity and discontinuity of attachment from infancy through adolescence. *Child Development*, 71, 690–694.

Hardy, T. (2004). *Tess of the d'Urbevilles*. Ann Arbor, MI: Borders Classics.

Hass, E., Hill, R., Lambert, M. J., & Morrell, B. (2002). Do early responders to psychotherapy maintain treatment gains? *Journal of Clinical Psychology*, 58, 1157–1172.

Haynes, B., Deveraux, P., & Guyatt, G. (2002). Physicians' and patients' choices in evidence-based practice: Evidence from within: A new paradigm for clinical practice does not make decisions, people do. *British Medical Journal*, *324*, 1350.

Healy, D. (2005). *Psychiatric drugs explained*. New York: Elsevier.

Henry, W. P., Schacht, T. E., Strupp, H. H., Butler, S. F., & Binder, J. L. (1993). Effects of training in time-limited psychotherapy: Mediators of therapist's responses to training. *Journal of Consulting and Clinical Psychology*, *61*, 441–447.

Hill, C. E., & Lambert, M. J. (2004). Methodological issues in studying psychotherapy processes and outcomes. In M. J. Lambert (Ed.), *Bergin and Garfield's handbook of psychotherapy and behavior change* (5th ed., pp. 72–114). New York: Wiley.

Hilsenroth, M. (2007). A programmatic study of short-term psychodynamic psychotherapy: Assessment, process, outcome, and training. *Psychotherapy Research*, *17*, 31–45.

Hoffman, I. (1998). *Ritual and spontaneity in the psychoanalytic process: A dialectical-constructivist view*. Hillsdale, NJ: Analytic Press.

Hollon, S. D. (1996). The efficacy and effectiveness of psychotherapy relative to medication. *American Psychologist*, *51*, 1025–1030.

Hollon, S. (2006). Randomized clinical trials. In J. Norcross, L. Beutler, & R. Levant (Eds.), *Evidence based practices in mental health* (pp. 96–104). Washington, DC: American Psychological Association Press.

Hollon, S. D., Thase, M. E., & Markowitz, J. C. (2002). Treatment and prevention of depression. *Psychological Science in the Public Interest*, 3, 39–77.

Horney, K. (1937). *The neurotic personality of our time*. New York: Norton.

Howard, K. I., Cornille, T., Lyons, J., Vessey, J., Leuger, R., & Saunders, S. (1996). Patterns of mental health service utilization. *Archives of General Psychiatry*, 53, 696–703.

Hunsley, J. (2007). Addressing key challenges in evidence-based practice in psychology. *Professional Psychology: Research and Practice*, 39, 113–121.

Hurt, S., Reznikoff, M., & Clarkin, J. (1991). *Psychological assessment, psychiatric diagnosis, treatment planning*. New York: Brunner/Mazel.

Institute of Medicine. (2001). *Crossing the quality chasm: A new health system for the 21st century*. Washington, DC: National Academy Press.

Inui, T. S., & Frankel, R. M. (2006). Hello, stranger: Building a healing narrative that includes everyone. *Academic Medicine, 81*, 415–418.

Jacobson, N. S., & Christensen, A. (1996a). *Integrative couple therapy: Promoting acceptance and change*. New York: Norton.

Jacobson, N. S., & Christensen, A. (1996b). Studying the effectiveness of psychotherapy: How well can clinical trials do the job? *American Psychologist, 51*, 1031–1039.

Jones, E. E., & Pulvos, S. M. (1993). Comparing the process in psychodynamic and cognitive-behavioral therapies. *Journal of Consulting and Clinical Psychology, 61*, 306–316.

Jung, C. G. (1975). The theory of psychoanalysis. In *Critique of psychoanalysis* (pp. 92–156). Princeton, NJ: Princeton University Press. (Original work published 1913)

Kagan, J. (1997). Conceptual psychopathology: The importance of developmental profiles. *Development and Psychopathology*, 9, 221–234.

Kendall, P. C. (1999). Clinical significance. *Journal of Consulting and Clinical Psychology*, 67, 283–284.

Kendall, P. C., & Chambless, D. L. (Eds.). (1998). Empirically supported psychological therapies. *Journal of Consulting and Clinical Psychology*, 66, 3–167.

Kennedy, T., Regehr, G., & Rosenfeld, J. (2004). Exploring the gap between knowledge and behavior: A qualitative study of clinician action following an educational intervention. *Academic Medicine, 79*, 386–393.

Kihlstrom, J. F. (1998). If you've got an effect, test its significance: If you've got a weak effect, do a meta-analysis (Commentary on "Precis of statistical significance: Rationale, validity, and utility" by S. L. Chow). *Behavioral and Brain Sciences, 21*, 205–206.

Kihlstrom, J. F., & Kihlstrom, L. C. (1998). Integrating science and practice in an environment of managed care. In D. K. Routh & R. J. DeRubeis (Eds.), *The science of clinical psychology: Accomplishments and future directions* (pp. 281–293). Washington, DC: American Psychological Association.

Klein, M. (1957). *Envy and gratitude*. New York: Basic Books.

Krueger, R. E. (1999). The structure of common mental disorders. *Archives of General Psychiatry*, 56, 921–926.

Kreuger, R. E., & Piasecki, T. M. (2002). Toward a dimensional and psychometrically-informed approach to conceptualizing psychopathology. *Behavior Research and Therapy*, 40, 485–499.

Krupnick, J. L., Sotsky, S. M., Simmens, S., Moyer, J., Elkin, I., Watkins, J., et al. (1996). The role of the therapeutic alliance in psychotherapy and pharmacotherapy outcomes: Findings in the National Institute of Mental Health Treatment of Depression Collaborative Research Program. *Journal of Consulting and Clinical Psychology*, 64, 532–539.

Kubiszyn, T., Meyer, G., Finn, S., Eyde, L., Kay, G., Moreland, K., et al. (2000). Empirical support for psychological assessment in clinical health care settings. *Professional Psychology: Search and Practice, 31*, 119–130.

Kuhn, T. S. (1962). *The structure of scientific revolutions*. Chicago: University of Chicago Press.

Laing, R. D. (1965). *The divided self*. Baltimore: Pelican. (Original work published 1959)

Lambert, M. (2004). *Bergin and Garfield's handbook of psychotherapy and behavioral change*. New York: Wiley.

Lambert, M. (2007). Presidential address: What we have learned from a decade of research aimed at improving psychotherapy outcome in routine care. *Psychotherapy Research, 17*, 1–14.

Lambert, M., Whipple, J., Hawkins, E. Vermeesch, D., Nielson, S., & Smart, D. (2003). Is it time for clinicians routinely to track patient outcome? A meta-analysis. *Clinical Psychology, 10*, 299–301.

Lamporpoulos, G. K., Goldfried, M. R., Castonguay, L. G., Lambert, M. J., Stiles, W. B., & Nestoros, J. N. (2002). What kind of research can we realistically expect from the practitioner? *Journal of Clinical Psychology, 58*, 1241–1264.

Levant, R. E. (2004). The empirically validated treatment: A practitioner/educator perspective. *Clinical Psychology: Science and Practice, 11*, 219–224.

Levenson, E. (1998). Awareness, insight, and learning. *Contemporary Psychoanalysis, 34*, 239–249.

Levine, M. (2006). *The price of privilege: How parental pressure and material advantage are creating a generation of unhappy kids*. New York: HarperCollins.

Lidz, T. (1968). *The person: His development throughout the life cycle*. New York: Basic Books.

Linehan, M. M. (1993). *Cognitive-behavioral treatment of borderline personality disorder*. New York: Guilford Press.

Lipkin, M., Putnam, S., & Lazare, A. (Eds.). (1995). *The medical interview*. New York: Springer-Verlag.

Lipsey, M. W., & Wilson, D. B. (1993). The efficacy of psychological, educational, and behavioral treatment: Confirmation from meta-analysis. *American Psychologist, 48*, 1181–1209.

Luborsky, L. (1984). *Principles of psychoanalytic psychotherapy: A manual for supportive-expressive treatment*. New York: Basic Books.

Luborsky, L., & Crits-Cristoph, P. (1990). *Understanding transference: The CCRT method (the core conflictual relationship theme)*. New York: Basic Books.

Luborsky, L., Diguer, L., Seigman, D. A., Rosenthal, R., Krause, E. D., Johnson, S., et al. (1999). The researcher's own therapy allegiances: A "wild card" in comparisons of treatment efficacy. *Clinical Psychology: Science and Practice, 6*, 95–106.

Luborsky, L., McLellan, A., Woody, G., O'Brian, C., & Auerbach, A. (1985). Therapist success and its determinants. *Archives of General Psychiatry, 42*, 602–611.

Mahler, M. (1972). On the first three sub-phases of the separation individuation process. *International Journal of Psychoanalysis, 53*, 333–338.

Malik, M., Alimohamed, S., Holoway, R., & Beutler, L. (2000, June). *Are all cognitive therapies alike? Validation of the TPRS*. Paper presented at the annual meeting of the Society for Psychotherapy Research, Chicago, IL.

Maruish, M. F. (Ed.). (1999). *The use of psychological testing for treatment planning and outcome assessment* (2nd ed.). Mahwah, NJ: Lawrence Erlbaum Associates.

Maruish, M. F. (2002). *Essentials of treatment planning*. New York: Wiley.

Maser, J., Kaelber, C., & Weise, R. (1991). International use and attitudes toward the DSM III and DSM III R: Growing consensus in psychiatric classification. *Journal of Abnormal Psychology, 100*, 271–279.

Meyer, G. J. (Ed.). (2001). Special section II: The utility of the Rorschach for clinical assessment II. *Psychological Assessment, 13*, 419–502.

Meyer, G. J. (2003). The reliability and validity of the Rorschach and Thematic Apperception Test (TAT) compared to other psychological and medical procedures: An analysis of systematically gathered evidence. In M. Hersen (Series Ed.) & M. Hilsenroth & D. Segal (Vol. Eds.), *Comprehensive handbook of psychological assessment: Vol. 3. Personality assessment* (pp. 315–342). Hoboken, NJ: Wiley.

Meyer, G., Finn, S., Eyde, L., Kay, G., Moreland, K., Dies, R., et al. (2001). Empirical support for psychological assessment in clinical health care settings. *Professional Psychology: Research and Practice, 31*, 119–130.

Meyer, G. J., Finn, S. E., Eyde, L. D., Kay, G. G., Moreland, K. L., Dies, R. R., et al. (2001). Psychological testing and psychological assessment: A review of evidence and issues. *American Psychologist, 56*, 128–165.

Miller, S. J., & Binder, J. L. (2002). The effects of manual-based training on treatment fidelity and outcome. A review of the literature on adult individual psychotherapy. *Psychotherapy, 39*, 184–198.

Millon, T. (1996). *Disorders of personality: DSM IV and beyond*. New York: Wiley.

Mischler, E. (1979). Meaning in context: Is there any other kind? *Harvard Educational Review, 49*(1), 1–19.

Mischler, E. (1984). *The discourse of medicine: Dialectics of medical interviews*. Norwood, NJ: Ablex.

Mischler, E. G., & Clark, J. A. (1989). The language of attentive patient care: A comparison of two medical interviews. *Journal of General Internal Medicine*, 4(4), 325–335.

Mitchell, S. (1997). *Influence and autonomy in psychoanalysis*. Hillsdale, NJ: Analytic Press.

Mitchell, S. (1998). The analyst's knowledge and authority. *Psychoanalytic Quarterly*, 68, 1–31.

Morey, L.C. (1988). Personality disorders in DSM-III and DSM-III-R: An examination of convergence, coverage, and internal consistency. *American Journal of Psychiatry, 145*, 573–577.

Morgan, D., & Morgan, R. (2003). Single-participant research design: Bringing science to managed care. In A. Kazdin (Ed.), *Methodological issues and strategies in clinical research* (3rd ed., pp. 635–654). Washington, DC: American Psychological Association.

Morrow-Bradley, C., & Elliot, R. (1986). The utilization of psychotherapy research by practicing psychotherapists. *American Psychologist, 41*, 188–197.

Mueller, T. I., Leon, A., & Keller, M. (1999). Recurrence after recovery from major depressive disorder during 15 years of observational follow-up. *American Journal of Psychiatry, 156*, 1000–1006.

Najavits, L. M., & Strupp, H. H. (1994). Differences in the effectiveness of psychodynamic therapies: A process-outcome study. *Psychotherapy, 31*(1), 114–123.

Nathan, P. E., & Gorman, J. M. (Eds.). (1998). *A guide to treatments that work.* New York: Oxford University Press.

Nierenberg, A. (1994). The treatment of severe depression: Is there an efficacy gap between the SSRI and TCA antidepressant generations? *Journal of Clinical Psychopharmacology, 14*, 55–61.

Norcross, J. C. (Ed.). (2002). *Psychotherapy relationships that work: Therapist contributions and responsiveness to patients' needs.* New York: Oxford University Press.

Norcross, J. C., Beutler, L. E., & Levant, R. F. (2002). *Evidence-based practices in mental health.* Washington, DC: American Psychological Association.

Ogden, T. (1982). *Projective identification and psychotherapeutic technique.* Northvale, NJ: Jason Aronson.

Ogden, T. (1986). *The matrix of the mind: Object relations and the psychoanalytic dialogue.* Northvale, NJ: Jason Aronson.

Ogles, B. M., Lambert, M. J., & Sawyer, J. D. (1995). Clinical significance of the National Institute of Mental Health Treatment of Depression Collaborative Research Program data. *Journal of Consulting and Clinical Psychology, 63*, 321–326.

Ollendick, T. H., & King, N. J. (2004). Empirically supported treatments for children and adolescents: Advances toward evidence-based practice. In P. M. Barrett & T. H. Ollendick (Eds.), *Handbook of interventions that work with children and adolescents: Prevention and treatment* (pp. 3–26). New York: Wiley.

Parry, G., Cape, J., & Pilling, S. (2003). Clinical practice guidelines in clinical psychology and psychotherapy. *Clinical Psychology and Psychotherapy, 10*, 337–351.

Phillips, L., & Andrews, R. (2001). Clinical inertia. *Annals of Internal Medicine, 118*, 825–834.

Piaget, J. (1954). *The construction of reality in the child.* New York: Basic Books. (Original work published 1937)

Pinquart, M., Duberstein, P., & Lyness, J. (2006). Treatments for later life depressive conditions: A meta-analytic comparison of pharmacotherapy and psychotherapy. *American Journal of Psychiatry, 163*, 1403–1502.

Pinsky, R. (1976). *The situation of poetry.* Princeton, NJ: Princeton University Press.

Plunkin, E. (2006, June 1). Psychotherapy in the age of the brain. *Psychiatric Times*, 62–68.

Reiser, R., & Thompson, L. W. (2005). *Bipolar disorder: Advances in psychotherapy—Evidence-based practice.* Cambridge, MA: Hogrefe & Huber.

Roth, A., & Fonagy, P. (2005). *What works for whom* (2nd ed.). New York: Guilford Press.

Rounsaville, B. J., Glazer, W., O'Malley, S., Foley, S., & Weissman, M. (1988). Role of manual guided training in the conduct and efficacy of interpersonal therapy for depression. *Journal of Consulting and Clinical Psychology*, *56*, 681–688.

Roussos, A., Lissin, L., & De Duarte, A. (2007). The importance of theoretical framework in the formulation of clinical inferences in psychotherapy. *Psychotherapy Research*, *17*, 535–543.

Sackett, D., Straus, S., Richardson, W., Rosenbert, W., & Haynes, R. (2000). *Evidence based medicine* (2nd ed.). London: Churchill Livingstone.

Sandell, R., Lazar, A., Grant, J., Carlsson, J., & Broberg, J. (2006). Therapists' therapies: The relation between training therapy and patient change in long-term psychotherapy and psychoanalysis. *Psychotherapy Research*, *16*, 306–316.

Schatzberg, A., Cole, J., & DiBattista, C. (2005). *Manual of clinical pharmacology*. Washington, DC: American Psychiatric Publishing.

Schwaber, E. (1996). Toward a definition of the term and concept of interaction: Its reflection in analytic listening. *Psychoanalytic Inquiry*, *16*, 5–24.

Settlage, C. (1992). Therapeutic process and developmental process in the restructuring of object and self constancy. *Journal of the American Psychoanalytic Association*, *41*, 473–492.

Sharpe, D. (1997). Of apples and oranges, file drawers and garbage: Why validity issues in meta-analysis will not go away. *Clinical Psychology Review*, *17*, 881–901.

Silberschatz, G. (2005). *Transformative relationships: The control-mastery theory of psychology*. New York: Routledge.

Skodol, M. (1988). Validating structured DSM-III-R personality disorder assessments with longitudinal data. *American Journal of Psychiatry*, *145*, 1297–1299.

Slavin, M., & Kriegman, D. (1998). Why the analyst needs to change: Toward a theory of conflict, negotiation and mutual influence in the therapeutic process. *Psychoanalytic Dialogues*, *8*, 247–284.

Smith, B., & Smith, D. (1995). *The Cambridge companion to Husserl*. Cambridge: Cambridge University Press.

Smith, M. L., & Glass, G. V. (1977). *Meta-analysis of psychotherapy outcome studies*. Baltimore: Johns Hopkins University Press.

Smith, M. L., Glass, G. V., & Miller, R. L. (1980). *The benefits of psychotherapy*. Baltimore: Johns Hopkins University Press.

Sroufe, L. A., Egeland, B., Carlson, E., & Collins, W. A. (2005). *The development of the person: The Minnesota Study of Risk and Adaptation from Birth to Adulthood*. New York: Guilford Press.

Stein, D. M., & Lambert, M. J. (1995). Graduate training in psychotherapy: Are therapy outcomes enhanced? *Journal of Consulting and Clinical Psychology*, *63*, 182–196.

Stein, D., Lerer, B., & Stahl, S. (2005). *Evidence-based psychopharmacology*. New York: Cambridge University Press.

Stewart, M., Brown, J., Donnar, A., McWhinney, A., Oates, J., Weston, W., et al. (2000). The impact of patient-centered care on patient outcomes. *Journal of Family Practice*, *49*, 796–804.

Stiles, W. B., Shapiro, D. A., & Elliot, R. (1986). Are all psychotherapies equivalent? *American Psychologist, 41*, 165–180.

Strauss, B. M., & Kaechele, H. (1998). The writing on the wall: Comments on the current discussion about empirically validated treatments in Germany. *Psychotherapy Research, 8*, 158–170.

Stuart, R., & Lilienfeld, S. (2007). The evidence missing from evidence-based practice. *American Psychologist, 62*, 615–616.

Sullivan, H. (1953). *The interpersonal theory of psychiatry*. New York: Norton.

Szasz, T. (1961). *The myth of mental illness*. New York: Harper & Row.

Tanenbaum, S. J. (2003). Evidence-based practice in mental health: Practical weaknesses meet political strengths. *Journal of Evaluation in Clinical Practice*, 9, 287–301.

Tanenbaum, S. J. (2005). Evidence-based practice as mental health policy: Three controversies and a caveat. *Health Affairs, 24*, 163–173.

Thomas, A., & Chess, S. (1980). *The dynamics of psychological development*. New York: Brunner/Mazel.

Wagner, H. (1970). *Alfred Schultz: On phenomenology and social relations*. Chicago: University of Chicago Press.

Wallerstein, R. (1992). Psychoanalytic pluralism. In *The common ground of psychoanalysis* (pp. 3–62). Northvale, NJ: Jason Aronson.

Wampold, B. E. (2001). *The great psychotherapy debate: Models, methods, and findings*. Mahwah, NJ: Lawrence Erlbaum Associates.

Wampold, B. E., & Bhati, K. S. (2004). Attending to the omissions: A historical examination of the evidence-based practice movement. *Professional Psychology: Research and Practice, 35*, 563–570.

Wampold, B., & Bolt, D. (2006). Therapist effects: Clever ways to make them (and everything else) disappear. *Psychotherapy Research, 16*, 184–187.

Watson, J. C., & Rennie, D. L. (1994). Qualitative analysis of clients' subjective experience of significant moments during the exploration of problematic reactions. *Journal of Counseling Psychology, 41*, 500–509.

Weinberger, J., & Westen, D. (2004). When clinical description becomes statistical prediction. *American Psychologist, 59*, 595–613.

Weiss, J. (1993). *How psychotherapy works: Process and technique*. New York: Guilford Press.

Westen, D., & Bradley, R. (2005). Empirically supported complexity: Rethinking evidence-based psychotherapy. *Current Directions in Psychological Science, 14*, 266–271.

Westen, D., Heim, A., Morrison, K., Patterson, M., & Campbell, L. (2002). Simplifying diagnosis using a prototype-matching approach: Implications for the next edition of the DSM. In L. E. Beutler & M. L. Malik (Eds.), *Rethinking the DSM: A psychological perspective* (pp. 221–250). Washington, DC: American Psychological Association.

Westen, D., Novotny, C., & Thompson-Brenner, H. (2004). The empirical status of empirically supported psychotherapies: Assumptions, findings, and reporting in controlled clinical trials. *Psychological Bulletin*, *130*, 631–663.

Yates, T., Dodds, M., Sroufe, L., & Egeland, B. (2003). Exposure to partner violence and child behavior problems. *Development and Psychopathology*, *15*, 199–218.

Author Index

Subject Index

About the Author

Steven Frankel, M.D., has been a practicing psychiatrist for over thirty years. A graduate of Yale University Medical School, he is board certified in both general and child psychiatry. He is an associate clinical professor at the University of California Medical School and founder and director of the Center for Collaborative Psychology and Psychiatry in Kentfield, California.

www.ingramcontent.com/pod-product-compliance
Ingram Content Group UK Ltd.
Pitfield, Milton Keynes, MK11 3LW, UK
UKHW012040150926
475560UK00001B/106

9 780765 705907